'Dr Shahnavaz is to be commended for writing such a useful book, especially during these times when the phenomenon of refugees is so prominent in our societies. It is unique because of its specific focus on couples and families and its systemic approach, examining the interactive implications of these forms of adversities. The inclusion of relevant clinical material brings to life the complexities of these painful realities, whilst it also indicates ways of effectively addressing them. The book will be a valuable resource both for specialists and for the general public.'

Renos K Papadopoulos, *PhD, Professor at the University of Essex, UK. Author of* Involuntary Dislocation: Home, Trauma, Resilience and Adversity-Activated Development *(Routledge, 2021)*

'An important and timely contribution to the clinical work with highly traumatized refugees and their families—very moving, personal and instructive! Essential reading for all practitioners listening to seemingly unspeakable narratives . . .'

Dr E. Asen, *Consultant Psychiatrist, University College London & Anna Freud National Centre for Children and Families, UK*

'At one level, Dr. Shahnavaz's honest new book is an academic text, with a comprehensive review of literature and an examination of the contemporary political and social contexts in which refugee lives are embedded. At the heart of the book are compelling real-life accounts of refugee couples' experiences and journeys, woven in with the author's reflexive experiences of migration. It is these narratives that transport the book from an academic text to a complex hybrid between historical biography and autobiography. The book is written in a lucid and accessible style and includes a helpful overview and critique of therapeutic interventions for refugee couples and families. It skillfully examines the controversial subject of whether cultural and linguistic matching between the family and therapist is necessary for the therapeutic relationship. The book is a "must read" for students and teachers of refugee studies; for clinicians working with refugees; for service providers and policy makers; for service users; and for all those who are interested in culture, couple and family relationships and the impact of transgenerational trauma.'

Dr Reenee Singh, *Consultant Family and Systemic Psychotherapist & Founding Director, London Intercultural Couples Centre at the Child and Family Practice, UK*

W0113626

Working Systemically with Refugee Couples and Families

This stirring and insightful book explores how family dynamics among refugees are affected by the trauma of forced migration.

Written by an experienced family therapist, it uses a systemic perspective to understand the impact on couple relationships and parenting, as well as the broader issue of cultural and social assimilation. Shedding light on the complex and relational nature of the trauma experienced by refugee families, including issues around gender and mental health, Shadi Shahnavaz examines the clinical implications for those who care for them. The unique, in-depth interviews with refugees provide a rare insight into their journey to England and the adverse experiences they encounter along the way. Rather than a simple reflection on practice, Shahnavaz invites the reader to think about the ways in which they can connect with others, even in challenging and unfamiliar situations.

Working Systemically with Refugee Couples and Families is essential reading for any therapist or counsellor working today.

Shadi Shahnavaz is a social worker and systemic therapist. She has worked for over 25 years with complex families and individuals and has extensive experience in working with refugees. Shahnavaz presents and provides training on attachment theory, working with trauma, and working systemically. She has her own private practice and is head of Children and Families Services in a London mental health service.

The Systemic Thinking and Practice Series
Series Editors: Charlotte Burck and Gwyn Daniel

This influential series was co-founded in 1989 by series editors David Campbell and Ros Draper to promote innovative applications of systemic theory to psychotherapy, teaching, supervision and organisational consultation. In 2011, Charlotte Burck and Gwyn Daniel became series editors and aim to present new theoretical developments and pioneering practice, to make links with other theoretical approaches, and to promote the relevance of systemic theory to contemporary social and psychological questions.

Recent titles in the series include:

For more information about this series, please visit: www.routledge.com.

Working Systemically with Refugee Couples and Families

Exploring Trauma, Resilience and Culture

Shadi Shahnavaz

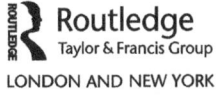

Routledge
Taylor & Francis Group

LONDON AND NEW YORK

Cover image: Benjamin Toth / Getty images

First published 2023
by Routledge
4 Park Square, Milton Park, Abingdon, Oxon OX14 4RN

and by Routledge
605 Third Avenue, New York, NY 10158

Routledge is an imprint of the Taylor & Francis Group, an informa business

British Library Cataloguing-in-Publication Data
A catalogue record for this book is available from the British Library

Library of Congress Cataloging-in-Publication Data
Names: Shahnavaz, Shadi, author.
Title: Working systemically with refugee couples and families:
  exploring trauma, resilience and culture / Shadi Shahnavaz.
Description: Abingdon, Oxon; New York, NY: Routledge, 2023. |
  Includes bibliographical references and index.
Identifiers: LCCN 2022008428 (print) | LCCN 2022008429 (ebook) |
  ISBN 9781032316529 (hardback) | ISBN 9780367416393 (paperback) |
  ISBN 9781003310716 (ebook)
Subjects: LCSH: Refugees—Mental health. | Refugee families—
  Mental health. | Forced migration—Psychological aspects. |
  Psychic trauma—Treatment.
Classification: LCC RC451.4.R43 S53 2023 (print) | LCC RC451.4.R43
  (ebook) | DDC 362.19689/0086914—dc23/eng/20220708
LC record available at https://lccn.loc.gov/2022008428
LC ebook record available at https://lccn.loc.gov/2022008429

ISBN: 978-1-032-31652-9 (hbk)
ISBN: 978-0-367-41639-3 (pbk)
ISBN: 978-1-003-31071-6 (ebk)

DOI: 10.4324/9781003310716

Typeset in Times New Roman
by Apex CoVantage, LLC

Contents

Series Editors' Foreword

The publication of this book could hardly be more timely. As the UK receives numbers of refugee families from Afghanistan, there is an ongoing need to expand our ways of understanding their cultural contexts, the particular types of adversity and trauma they have suffered, their fears for the safety and well-being of family left behind and the most effective ways of engaging with them and meeting their needs.

Despite much writing about the experiences of refugees, the legacy of trauma and the ongoing stresses of adaptation to host country, little has been written about the impact of these experiences on couple and family relationships, nor indeed on the multiple ways in which shared experiences may either lead to closeness and solidarity or to distance, withdrawal, secrecy and silence.

The great strength of Shadi Shahnavaz's book is that it attends in a sensitive and nuanced way to all these dimensions. Based on research interviews as well as on her own long experience of therapeutic work with Afghani and other Middle Eastern couples and families, the book enables the reader to connect at a profound level with the particular circumstances of each family she introduces. The in-depth interviews with four couples offer an invitation to engage with the complexity of their experiences at different stages—their circumstances in the home country, the hardship of the journey and the attempt to find a life within the UK. As a systemic therapist, Shadi is uniquely well placed to hold multiple narratives in mind while she listens to the individual—often shared for the first time—narratives of each of the participants. This provides the reader with multilayered testimonies which bring into focus the power of the individual story, the extent to which traumatic experiences, fears, vulnerabilities and anxieties may be hidden from—in some cases *especially* from—their most intimate family members. The need for therapists working in this context to be aware of all those experiences and emotions which may lie out of sight when they encounter refugee families is powerfully argued in this book, enhanced by Shadi's reflexive awareness of the connections with her own life experiences. She argues strongly for the importance of self-reflection in facing the horror and trauma that so many families have endured and the way such a personal engagement needs to underpin the creation of a space where clients can say the unsayable.

The book provides many perceptive angles on the literature about refugee experiences, trauma, resilience and culture, demonstrating the need to avoid simplistic categorisations and to pay attention to the specifics of human experience, the nuances of cultural experience and the complexities of family relationships. Shadi opens readers' eyes to the gulf that may emerge between a therapist's ideas about what is helpful to refugees and refugees' own ideas and experiences. The need to pay attention to power relations, especially in cultural contexts where giving direct feedback to those in authority would not be deemed appropriate, is helpfully developed in this book, as is the sensitivity many refugees might feel about not overwhelming therapists with their traumatic experiences and their acute vigilance to matters of being misunderstood, judged or abandoned.

Another feature of the book is that it also contains interviews with people working with refugees so that the complexities of the encounters, including the use of interpreters, are explored from different perspectives. There are helpful examples of the many misunderstandings, misreadings of cultural codes and disappointments that inevitably arise within this work.

Shadi's own therapeutic approach, in which she carefully and sensitively calibrates individual sessions, couples' meetings and sessions with children, will provide the reader with many ideas to enhance their own practice. She emphasises the importance of taking time and provides much wisdom about the need to go at the family's pace. She also describes how necessary it is to have a solid trusting relationship with parents in order to helpfully engage with children.

Above all, in this book, Shadi invites us alongside her on a journey into human suffering, where she manages to remain open hearted, hopeful, committed and steadfast and, in the process, inspires the reader to likewise find courage and hold onto hope and confidence.

We are delighted to include this book in our series.

Charlotte Burck
Gwyn Daniel

February 2022

Introduction

Although many authors have written about refugees and forced migration, and the effects of trauma on them as individuals (James, 2010; Kohli, 2007; Papadopoulos, 2021), very little has been written about the effects of traumatic experiences on refugee couples and families, looking at interactions within families and the part they play in the processing of traumatic experiences.

There are two parts to this book; in the first section I present an in-depth understanding of the experiences of refugees who have suffered trauma and their needs, in their own words, drawing on material from interviews with refugee participants. The book brings new insight into the impact of trauma on couple relationships and on parents' relationships with their children, with couples speaking profoundly about their changed parenting capacities and how their adverse experiences affected family dynamics. As a family therapist–researcher I held the individual's various roles in mind during our conversations to make connections between their roles as parents, as part of a couple and as individuals who themselves belong to families they had been forced to leave behind.

In the second section I examine help offered to refugees and refugee families. I draw on my own clinical experience of working with refugees and include material from other professionals' work with refugees. I discuss the clinical implications of the challenges faced by health services in meeting the mental health needs of non-Western individuals. In this book I refer to my work with refugees from the Middle East. With the large influx of Afghani refugees to the UK, I hope this book gives more insight into how to work with this population. The Afghanis have recently been re-traumatised by the Taliban re-taking control of the country, as a consequence of the withdrawal of NATO forces. After having held onto hope during the last 20 years when things were progressing in Afghanistan, many Afghan refugees had a yearning of returning to their home country; with the recent events they now feel depleted and empty. Refugees trying to enter the UK will have lost everything and possibly had to leave beloved family members behind, as well as losing their home and their safety. They will need a great deal of support to heal and connect with the Afghani community already in the UK.

This is not a standard academic text, nor one which simply looks at practice. It invites the reader to reach within themselves to think about how they might

DOI: 10.4324/9781003310716-1

connect even in circumstances where connection might seem unlikely—and to reflect on the time they might need in order to do this. I hope practitioners can have a better understanding of the importance of moving at the clients' pace and learning to witness their stories over and over again in a healing process.

This is a book which will give insight into the impact of trauma on individuals and their relationships with close family members as well as the larger society, from the point of view of the refugees themselves, and will open up ways of working with individuals and their families which keep relationships as their focus. I hope to demonstrate the importance of empathic listening as well as providing a containing environment so that refugee families can build trust. I aim to show how crucial it is in working with refugees to be able to be self-reflective in the context of such horror and trauma. These are all important aspects of creating a space where refugee clients feel that they can say the unsayable and that they will be heard and not judged.

References

James, K. (2010), Domestic Violence within Refugee Families: Intersecting Patriarchal Culture and the refugee Experience. *The Australian and New Zealand Journal of Family Therapy*, 31.

Kohli, R. (2007), *Social Work with Unaccompanied Asylum Seeking Children*. London: Palgrave Macmillan.

Papadopoulos, R.K. (2021), *Involuntary Dislocation: Home*. London: Trauma, Resilience, and Adversity-Activated Development, Routledge.

Chapter 1

My Background

Refugees live with the distress of not having a home they are welcomed into and, on a daily basis, experience the unwanted-ness they represent to the society they have been forced to seek refuge in for their survival. They therefore not only suffer from past adverse experiences but also live through traumas in the host country. I have been aware of this through my work as a family therapist in the NHS for many years, and I have been pained by the injustice of refugees' lives and situations.

In my earlier professional years, I worked as a social worker in Sweden and was saddened at how educated refugees from countries such as Iran and Iraq were not given the opportunity to use their expertise in Swedish society because of bureaucratic obstacles. Later, I worked as a social worker and family therapist in France and was again confronted with the integration difficulties of refugees from North African and sub-Saharan countries in France. Over the last 15 years I have worked in London with refugees from the Middle East especially, as our cultures have many similarities. Witnessing how affected these refugees were by their adverse experiences, I became interested in how their various traumas affected them as families and how relationships were impacted by their past and current sufferings. I decided to embark on a research study and interviewed refugee families with whom I did not work and did not know so that their experiences could help inform the development of our clinical work; this book is a result of the study. My personal story of forced migration has undoubtedly made me sensitive to the lived experiences of others who are forced to leave everything they are familiar with and call 'home', and readapt to a new, often hostile society. What is happening today with refugees trying to get into Greece from Turkey, for example, and being hit and cursed at by the local people and the Greek officials is an indication of the hostility refugees often face.

I am originally from Iran and moved to England when I was six years old as my father was studying for his doctorate in England. When I was ten, we moved back to Tehran in the hope of living there permanently. I had a big, loving family around me and lived a very comfortable life; I went to an international school where I had friends from all over the world, and I spent the best years of my life in the time I was allowed to live in my country. The revolution (1979) took it all

DOI: 10.4324/9781003310716-2

away, however, and I was obliged to leave my home, and all that went with it, just after my 13th birthday and a week before the Iran–Iraq War broke out. I remember queueing for days on end in front of the French embassy in the hope of obtaining a visa, praying nervously that they would welcome us. My maternal grandparents had both studied in Paris, and we therefore had a long history with France. They had bought a flat in Paris, which helped us in obtaining a visa. My father had left earlier than us and had gone to Germany in the hope of starting anew, as he had done most of his studies there; now it was our turn to leave, my mother, my older brother and me. My father was immediately offered a job as a lecturer at a university in Northern Sweden where he later was given a professorship (at the time he was in the newspapers because he was the first 'foreigner' to have become a professor in Sweden).

Leaving Iran was the saddest experience of my life, and I realise now, as an adult, how very low I had been for many years. My brother always said we were the 'lost' generation because in the years when we were supposed to be carefree and rebellious, we were too busy trying to adapt to a new way of life, new culture, new language and were isolated and far from our loved ones. When leaving our country, we were only allowed a suitcase each and everything else was left behind. My parents both went to live in Sweden and decided that it would be too disruptive for my brother and I to have to go to Sweden and learn a new language straight away after all the loss and upheaval we had experienced. They therefore left us to live with our maternal grandparents in Paris, where we went to a bilingual school. Soon, however, my very wise grandmother realised how unhappy I was and told my parents that my brother and I needed to be with them and adapt to Sweden as soon as possible.

I then lived ten tranquil years in Sweden, where I finished my university studies, before I moved back to Paris, where I always felt my roots to be.

During the time I was in Sweden my grandfather was arrested in Iran because they mistakenly thought he was a communist, and he was later released with an apology. My grandparents both aged many years in the months of his imprisonment, and my grandfather was never completely the same. Although I was never a refugee, I have lived through a great deal of loss and forced change; I believe this is why I have always been so interested in peoples' lives, especially refugees and their stories. When working with refugees I can relate to their sense of loss and pain and to their need to talk about their past lives in their home country. In the interviews with refugee couples, they all reflected how easy it had been for them to express themselves and open up about their experiences and their feelings because they knew I could understand them given our cultural similarities. When I say I was not a refugee it is because I went from one comfortable home to another through just one airplane ride. I had the security of having a visa which allowed me access to the country I was moving to and my father had a job with the same status as when we lived in Iran, so my social status did not change and we were not subjected to a profound upheaval in relation to family roles. Since we lived in Sweden and everyone speaks fluent

English there, I never needed to translate for my parents or to take on a different role than their daughter. I did not go through fear and anguish of the unknown like refugees, and I felt welcomed to the host country; I felt safe, but I suffered from a great deal of loss and forced change, and that is what I have in common with my refugee patients.

Chapter 2

The Effects of Trauma on Families

At the outset I would like to clarify that I deliberately use a somewhat specific definition of 'trauma'——namely, the state of mind and body as defined by the symptoms of Post-Traumatic Stress Disorder (PTSD). All of us will, of course, react with fight or flight when faced with adversity and extremely stressful situations. However, I speak of a person suffering from trauma when he/she/they continue to be hyper-alert and vigilant even when safe; although the person is no longer in danger, he/she/they continue to use the same self-protective coping strategies that they employed to protect themselves from psychological and emotional harm at the time of the traumatic experience. Hyper-vigilance, dissociation and avoidance are examples of coping strategies that may have been effective at the time of the traumatic experience but later interfere with the person's ability to live the life she/he/they want. The intrusion of the past into the present is one of the main problems confronting the trauma survivor; this intrusion may present as distressing intrusive memories, flashbacks, nightmares or overwhelming emotional states.

In the *Diagnostic and Statistical Manual of Mental Disorders, Fifth Edition* (*DSM-5*) the three-factor model of PTSD has been replaced by a four-factor model consisting of the following criteria: B) intrusion symptoms, C) persistent avoidance, D) altercations in cognition and mood and E) hyperarousal and reactivity symptoms. All *DSM-IV* PTSD symptoms have been retained in the *DSM-5*, and three new symptoms have been added: erroneous self- or other blame regarding the trauma; pervasive negative mood states involving fear, anger, guilt, shame, etc.; and reckless or self-destructive behaviour. The *DSM-IV* 'irritability' has become *DSM-5* 'aggressive behaviour'.

I find the definition of PTSD in *The International Classification of Diseases* (*ICD-11*) very helpful: This disorder follows exposure to an extremely threatening or horrific event or series of events. It consists of three core elements:

A) Re-experiencing: vivid intrusive memories, flashbacks or nightmares that involve re-experiencing in the present, accompanied by fear or horror. B) Avoidance: marked internal avoidance of thoughts and memories or external avoidance of activities or situations reminiscent of the traumatic event(s). C) Hyperarousal: a state of perceived current threat in the form of hyper-vigilance or an enhanced startle reaction. The symptoms interfere with normal functioning.

DOI: 10.4324/9781003310716-3

In this chapter I shall be sharing my experience of working with refugees and asylum seekers, looking deeper into some recurrent themes I have noticed both in my work in the field and in the interviews I had with the refugee couples. I shall be connecting with what other professionals have written on these matters, as well as drawing on other theoretical frameworks, such as psychoanalysis or attachment theory, because as a systemic practitioner, I am open to drawing upon other relevant approaches as well. I shall present each couple I interviewed in detail in the next chapter and give you the opportunity to hear their voices as they recount their experiences. My background as a family therapist leads me to hold in mind systemic complexities such as the relational nature of the events' impact on my participants' family members, as well as the effects of the wider societal discourses which colour the meaning, emphasis and quality of the lived experiences. I hold in mind the importance of the political at all levels: country of origin, familial contexts, host countries' policies and practices because each of these will impact on the couple and family relationships. We are relational human beings and are influenced by the context we live in.

Vulnerability

Almost all refugees and asylum seekers I work with express feeling vulnerable and helpless. Although their strength and resilience are often poignantly clear to me, they themselves convey a sense of helplessness and seem unconvinced when anyone tries to point out their achievements. This sense of helplessness is also apparent in the interviews I share in Chapter 3.

In my experience, refugees who have not been politically active in their home country often have more of a sense of vulnerability than those who have chosen to fight for their political convictions. It seems that an effect of being politically active is that of feeling more in control and of maintaining a sense of agency. Often, having the same political convictions can help a couple to feel more united, having a shared goal; this is clear, for example, in the documentary which won an Oscar in 2020, called *For Sama* about a couple in Syria and their fight for their beliefs.

Woodcock (2001) points out that families may either have a history of resistance or of being hapless bystanders who were swept up in the conflict. This will shape how they construct the meaning of what has befallen them. In my experience, refugees who are politically active seem to have more control, they know the risks they are taking and seem to be able to accept the consequences. Refugees who are victims of oppression and of simply being in the wrong place at the wrong time may be affected by their experiences of cruelty in a very different way; the sense of injustice stays with them for a long time after they are safe.

Secrets and Silence

This theme will become more apparent in the interviews I have shared in Chapter 3. Refugees must often keep their activities and whereabouts secret from friends and family members when they are in their home country, as no one can be trusted. When they decide to leave their country, it is most often in a clandestine manner, so the secrecy continues. In my experience, this secrecy then often turns into silence once the family is in the host country, silence between the family members. I shall go more deeply into the meanings and reasons for this silence in Chapter 4.

Vangelisti and Caughlin (1997) suggest that taboos and secrets generally represent vulnerabilities which, if revealed, could have relatively serious ramifications. In my work with refugee families, I have also seen that secrets can play a crucial and protective role for the couple; however, they do often lead to distancing and destruction in the relationship. Habitually when one partner has been tortured in prison, for example, they keep their experiences hidden from their companion to protect the image the other has of them, to shield the couple and the mutual respect, to not overstep boundaries. However, when the other partner is unaware of what his/her spouse has been through, there is a taboo there which creates distance and misunderstandings, leading to lack of mutual support and even more detachment. This becomes a vicious cycle, which in turn affects the children as well; they may either try to play the role of protectors by distracting the parents into having a shared goal (i.e. their children's problems), or isolate themselves from the parents and move towards friends outside of the family.

Papadopoulos (2002) offers a more positive appraisal for the presence of silence in refugee families. He describes how, through forced migration, people lose their home and their sense of belonging; that there are losses both in the inner and outer worlds of the refugees. Papadopoulos explains that while the outside changes are often sudden, the transitions to adjusting to these changes can be prolonged. In this context, Papadopoulos suggests that refugees are sometimes purposefully silent and that the silence allows them to heal over time. Papadopoulos goes on to explain that forced migration leaves people temporarily disoriented, as if frozen; a type of 'psychological hypothermia' and that they need to thaw out in order to proceed again to ordinary living. The silence in refugees can therefore be seen as having a protective factor, rather than a pathological one, as it allows the refugees space to reflect on their experiences and make sense of them in order to then be able to move on in their new environment. According to Papadopoulos, in the state of 'frozenness' (Papadopoulos and Hildebrand 1997) an individual, family and community limit their activity to the bare essentials and conserve energy, which helps them develop a reflective and meditative stance. However, I must say that from a systemic point of view, although silence can be therapeutic and helpful on an individual level, it can create distance and separation within the family. If each member suffers on their own and there is no sharing of thoughts, feelings and expressed emotions, the silence can become a heavy burden to carry for the children in the family, who often want to move on faster and adapt to their new life but may feel weighed down by the silence and all the unsaid.

On the other hand, the silence can also be seen as showing sensitivity and respect to each other in a family, where the couple does not want to burden each other or the children with their anxieties and suffering. Children are, however, rarely unaware of or protected from their parents' suffering; they just receive clear messages not to communicate their feelings and thoughts in the family, leaving them feeling confused, isolated and often self-blaming.

Kohli (2009) speaks about unaccompanied minors' reluctance to talk openly about their past lives, and the protective role that silence plays in their lives, both on the journey to safety and mostly in the country where they seek asylum. He means that the emergence and maintenance of silence and secrets can be seen as part of a process of healing, as well as a way of concealing and managing the confusion and disorder generated by forced migration. Kohli (2009) goes on to say that when unaccompanied minors do talk, they sometimes do so reluctantly and cautiously, with mistrust. My experience tells me that this can also apply to adults in refugee families, where there is less trust amongst family members, less of a sense that they can rely on one another to be helpful and strong, as they each know how fragile the other is.

Melzak (1992) and Woodcock (2001), speak about how sometimes in refugee families, the death of a parent is hidden from a child, to prevent the child developing beliefs that they were responsible for the death of the parent (Melzak, 1992). Having worked within the Iranian and Kurdish community, Ahlberg (2007) is also very aware of the cultural tendency to keep things unsaid. Ahlberg gives the example of the Iranian screenplay ('GAV', which means cow) of the 1970s, based on a novel by Gholam Hossein Saedi (an Iranian writer). The novel tells the complex story about a man who has gone mad because of a missing cow, and because well-intentioned neighbours had protected him from the truth about its death. There is a code of silence regarding certain particularly difficult or shameful problems, within the family and also with regard to outsiders (such as therapists). Ahlberg (2007) suggests that this difference in culture, where in the Western world it is believed it is best to talk about things more openly, may explain why it has often taken such a long time for a working alliance to develop with Farsi-speaking clients. In my work with refugees from Afghanistan, Kurdistan and Arab countries such as Iraq and Syria, I have come to recognise the value in the time it takes to build a trusting relationship. This may be due to the mistrust of professionals from other cultures and the interpreters they use. I have noticed that once they realise I understand their culture and the way family 'works' in their (our) culture and that my curiosity about their culture is genuine and non-judgemental, they open up and then the alliance becomes strong; that is when change can happen. This theme will be explored further in subsequent chapters.

Knudsen (1990, 1993) also views this under-communication of personal problems amongst refugees as a type of coping mechanism. Knudsen writes that refugees find silence a far better strategy than talking when they are in exile and in a situation which is beyond their control. There is another layer of complexity in my opinion where Iranians, Afghanis and Kurds often speak in code, things are not spoken about directly and one has to read between the lines. For this, one needs to have a deep cultural understanding, or the help of a very skilled interpreter. I cannot comment on whether my clients from Arab countries speak in code, as often the interpreter will translate in a way that makes sure I understand their meaning, so he/she may take away the subtleties.

Secrecy and Isolation

The silence which seems to have slowly made its way into the lives of the refugee families I work with, has not only created distance and separation between the family members but has often led to the isolation of the families in the new community. I have found in my work with Farsi-speaking refugees that there is a great deal of mistrust amongst us, and the Farsi-speaking community is very split and divided. Kurds, Iranians and Afghanis do not really mingle, and even amongst themselves, Iranians are quite distant and weary of each other. Darvishpour (1994) asserts that the lack of trust is, according to his view, typical of Iranian interrelationships in exile: a fact that also counteracts any tendencies towards ghettoisation among Iranians as compared perhaps to other communities. Melzak (1992) also writes about her experience of working with refugees who are turned against each other and very mistrustful. She goes on to explain that this is a central characteristic of life in a repressive regime that is then mirrored in some communities in exile. Many refugees I work with speak of not trusting authorities in England and feeling persecuted by them, for example, by the job centre or housing. They feel that they are seen as liars (just like back in their own home country) and that their every move is being monitored. Hence, they feel persecuted and harassed by the English system as well. I know from experience that in many refugee camps Afghanis and Syrians have had to be separated because of conflict and tensions between the two nationalities; the Afghanis often feel like second-class refugees, as according to them so much focus is on the Syrian refugees and their needs. This will now, most likely, change with Afghanistan being the focus at the moment.

Woodcock (2001) argues that the absence of social and cultural frameworks in exile may exacerbate feelings of alienation. I believe this to be a very important element in the suffering of refugees I work with, who have not been able to mourn their losses but who also find themselves left to manage by themselves without the support of friends, family and a warm and compassionate community that they can trust. Blackwell and Melzak (2000) write about the factors which help ameliorate distressing experiences and the important link between a sense of belonging to a group or a community and the well-being of the refugee families. I have often seen how, despite their need for support and a sense of belonging, refugee families' distrust takes over and hinders any positive connections with others who suffer for much the same reasons. Smyth and Kum (2010) also speak of the importance of social networks for refugee families. They say that having been forced to leave their home country, refugees lose their social networks, usually without the chance to prepare for this or to find out how to build new social networks wherever they may arrive.

Castles et al. (2002) suggest that where restrictive rules and rigid systems confine immigrants to a passive role, integration can be particularly slow and incomplete.

They posit that minority groups should be supported in maintaining their culture and social identities. I would argue here that more important than maintaining their culture is integrating their culture with the culture of the country they have sought refuge in and finding a balance between their culture of origin and the new culture in which their children are being brought up—a process that can take many years and many compromises but that can benefit families who manage it. I believe this integration can only take place if the families feel that their way of living and their culture is being respected. When I worked with refugee families in France, the school system there insisted on the children speaking French in their homes, often with parents who hardly spoke much French at all! The logic behind this was that the children would integrate faster, as well as the family, if they all spoke French (and thereby took on the French culture). The reality is that this rigid and insensitive demand put the families in a defensive position because they felt attacked in their culture, their language, and their values, and forced to take on a culture they were not only unfamiliar with but felt threatened by.

In their model of integration, Ager and Strang (2004, 2008) consider the different forms of social relationship that are important to integration, using the concept of social capital to distinguish between three different forms of social connection or relationship. These are 'social bonds', which are connections within a community defined by, for example, ethnic, national or religious identity. 'social bridges', which are relationships with members of other communities; and 'social links', which means connections with institutions, including local and central government services. In my opinion, what is lacking in this concept is the issue of 'class' because even if Iranians, for example, have social bonds in their national and ethnic identity, there is a deep-rooted class system in Iran, which means that often Iranians are shy of mixing with other Iranians until they are certain of their family backgrounds and class. In my opinion, it is therefore essential to understand the whole societal and historic context and not just focus on culture when working with refugees and working cross-culturally.

Strang and Ager (2010) assert that integration depends on the complementary development of social bridges as well as social bonds to avoid the emergence of separate, very bonded, but disconnected communities (referred to as 'silos' by Cantle, 2005). They go on to suggest that strengthened connection with pre-existing communities (so-called host communities) need not be at the expense of the strong ties that bind co-ethnic and other forms of indigenous identification. The evidence of the importance of bonds as a source of emotional support, self-esteem and confidence (Losi and Strang, 2008; Vrecer, 2010) underpins the claim that strong bonding capital supports the development of bridging capital. Spicer's (2008) study on neighbourhoods brings this out more clearly. His analysis focuses on refugees' experiences of particular neighbourhoods (the particular potency of the neighbourhood for refugees is also confirmed by Atfield, Brahnbhatt and O'Toole (2007), in suggesting that some neighbourhoods are experienced as 'including' and others as 'excluding'. The excluding neighbourhood is one where local people are seen to be unfriendly and where there are few or no residents from co-ethnic communities.

In this situation refugees lack the confidence to build up language skills and local knowledge; instead, they grow increasingly fearful and isolated.

In another paper, Woodcock (2000), explains how trauma can be an experience which makes adults feel totally disconnected, alone and isolated. He says that it is as if the internal parent that is present within each individual, who nurtures and protects us and who provides the foundations of basic trust in us is shattered in the survivor of trauma. This, Woodcock (2000) means, can lead to the adult feeling parentless, and a sense that no one can truly understand what has happened to them. This is experienced as a terrifying existential loneliness. This disturbed attachment to one's own internal representations of self and others may help us to understand why many individuals find it hard to socialise in the aftermath of extreme events and explains why previously outgoing, pro-social people become withdrawn and socially anxious, no longer able to maintain relationships with others. I can see this evidenced in my interviews with refugee couples, who all described themselves as having been outgoing and sociable and who are now quite withdrawn from society and afraid of building new relationships. I also see it in my work with refugees where they self-isolate for protection and as the therapeutic work advances, they begin to risk being more social.

A vicious cycle can develop where the individuals and families feel misunderstood or not understood and isolated; they therefore go into their own shells more and take refuge in silence and a quiet suffering which leads to them being even more isolated and silent. This may in turn lead to refugees being seen by the host society as not wanting to integrate and thereby result in more hostilities.

Couples' Past Lives

Alcock (2003) writes that our earliest sensations, and certainly our memories, come from the smells and the sounds of home. We learn to recognise and make sense of tones of voice, behaviours, and gestures, of music and song, of food to mark special occasions, of dress as information. We are born into a culture that we absorb through every pore. When we are displaced into a new environment, the bewilderment and profound sense of dislocation can show itself in physical disease. The psychological sense of home that has been located in people or places, when lost, can feel like an exhaustion of parts of the self, and one's identity itself can feel threatened. I have often heard refugees I work with say that they feel confused and have lost their sense of judgement, what is right and what is wrong, who they can trust and not, and this creates a real sense of fear, as if you no longer have any solid ground to stand on. This sense of lost assertiveness means that they are uncertain about guiding their children through life in the new country as they are so unfamiliar with the school system, the health care system and so forth; children pick up on their parents' uncertainties and fears, and they lose trust in their parents, which has a detrimental impact on them emotionally and psychologically.

In *Therapeutic Care for Refugees*, Papadopoulos (2002) examines closely the notions of home and clearly defines differences between that actual loss of home as a place, and this inner depletion. He recognises that each individual will be affected by a range of factors, a unique combination of personal experiences, circumstances and psychological resources. 'Home' refers to a fundamental cluster of basic proto processes, needs and abilities that form a

> mosaic substratum on top of which we build our individual and collective identity. Therefore, the loss of home creates for refugees a deep sense of lack, of disorientation and absence which is not easily definable either in terms of its nature or its effects.
>
> (Papadopoulos, 2002: 17)

Alcock (2003) says that the idealisation of the home and the hope to return may help people to survive. To me, it seems that the hope of return is not always to the home but can also be to a past identity. Somehow it would seem that remembering who they were helped my participants to feel less inner depletion, as if remembering their past identity gave them hope that they could be that person or couple again. I often use this returning to their past identities with my refugee patients, and it gives them strength and a sense that, even for a short moment, they are not just a refugee but also a human being with a past that was one they had chosen; being able to go back to the internal world of the past is an invaluable resource. In this I join Birkett (2006), who says that although the refugee may have lost his/her world, they carry it internally. The refugees I interviewed all spoke spontaneously and in detail about their past life and world; this seemed to give them strength as they were taken back in time through their internal store of memories.

Some time ago, I was working with an Afghani woman refugee who had been referred to me for severe depression and psychotic episodes. Social services had become involved, and I had to argue strongly to convince them not to place her three children into local authority care for neglect. I used to have to go to her home and walk with her back to the office to make her feel safe in the streets and make sure she got out of the flat she would hide away in. She had been a teacher in Afghanistan and had been arrested and put into prison after the Taliban came to power. She used to walk with a hunched back like an old lady and looked down at the ground. One time, as we walked along together, I asked her to tell me about the students in her class back home, and as she started to recount her past self as a teacher, her back became more and more straight and she became tall and held the allure of a proud woman. As we walked past a shop window, I signalled to her to look at that beautiful woman who was her reflection. She cried in my arms as she remembered, even if it was for an instant, who she had been, and I reminded her that that woman was still in her, somewhere, and that we would re-discover her together.

However, what has also become evident in my work with refugees is that living in the past can hinder individuals from moving forward. I agree with Woodcock (2001) when he argues that continued political resistance may signal a healthy desire to continue to struggle with realistic or idealistic aims; but it may also be the individual's inability to let go and to mourn the passing of a way of life and all the physical and emotional losses of exile. In my experience, if the myth of return becomes too dominant in the refugee's life, it can hinder the individual/family from adapting to their new situation. If one is always looking back and longing to go back to the past, one cannot or is not willing to move forward because the past is more certain than the future; we all know what we have left behind, good and bad, and if the present is difficult and the future is uncertain, it can be all too tempting to get stuck in the comfort of the past.

Resilience/Resistance

I would like to use Wade's (1997: 25) definition of resistance to illustrate my perception of resistance:

> any mental or behavioural act through which a person attempts to expose, withstand, repel, stop, prevent, abstain from, strive against, impede, refuse to comply with, or oppose any form of violence or oppression (including any type of disrespect), or the conditions that make such acts possible, may be understood as a form of resistance.
>
> (1997, p. 25)

Wade goes on to say that

> also any attempt to imagine or establish a life based on respect and equality, on behalf of one's self or others, including any effort to redress the harm caused by violence or other forms of oppression, represents a de facto form of resistance.
>
> (1997, p. 25)

To me, resilience and resistance go hand in hand because in order to resist the impact of oppression and adverse experience you have to be resilient, and resilience is in turn built up by the identification of acts of resistance. In the next chapter I will talk more about the resilience and resistance the couples I interviewed showed throughout their ordeals. Linking this to Woodcock's (2000) trauma and attachment theory, it would seem that most of my participants' 'internal parents' had strong roots and were able to protect and nurture them and help them show resilience at times of extreme difficulty. Indeed, in my clinical work I have seen a real connection between a person's strong attachment to their primary carer and their ability to be resilient in the face of adversity.

According to Alayarian (2007), resilient people are more often able to assess what needs to be dealt with: they tend to possess a good cognitive capacity and adequate emotional stability. For resilient people, things are seen as they are and are not easily dismissed; there is a clear distinction between fantasy and reality. She goes on to say that this enables them to respond more efficiently in difficult

situations and not be paralysed by anxiety. Alayarian (2007) also writes that resilient people are more aware and more tolerant of their negative feelings. Alayarian (2007) speaks of how resilient people are able to build a safe intra-psychic
space in which they live and talk to themselves to regulate pain. She says that
this almost unbreakable part of the self protects one from collapsing emotionally when the external world is unpredictable and life threatening. Alayarian does
warn that there is a fine line between being resilient on the one hand and repress-
ing one's feelings on the other hand.

It seems to me that the power to resist and to be resilient comes mostly from
love and care for others and strong political and moral convictions. Many studies have been carried out to show the importance of religious beliefs in coping
and gaining strength to be resilient (Bhui et al. 2008; Baasher, 2001; Cinnirella
and Loewenthal, 1999; Crossley, 1995; Dein, 2004; Esmail, 1996). I have often
thought that if many of the refugee families I work with did not have strong faith,
they would not have survived their ordeals. One family I am thinking of as I write
this is a family who, when they finally were given refugee status and a home,
lost their child to illness; they both said they felt that God had loved their child
so much that He had wanted him to join Him in paradise rather than to remain
on earth. This belief helped them to carry on fighting for a good life in England,
rather than to crumble with sorrow.

Jenkins (2011) speaks about 'ethical commitment' when speaking about one
of his clients, and this resonates strongly with my own experience of my clients,
many of whom showed resilience out of ethical commitment to their loved ones,
and others became resilient through their convictions of ethical commitment to
society, their fellow citizens, equality, political justice and freedom of speech.

Rutter (1985) outlines patterns of resilience and their acquisition, which in summary are the ability to integrate the traumatic experience in one's belief system;
the presence of self-esteem and the ability to be pro-active in the face of diverse
stresses; the presence of secure affectionate relationships; a measure of success
and achievement; the interaction with others in securing these gains; parental
modelling; the ability of the child to process events in a meaningful way; and
lastly, the ability to deal with stressful events, which in itself is a protective factor.
I would add to these qualities the humanity I have seen in my refugee clients and
the way they can still hold others in mind, even amongst the horror they are living
through. My refugee clients seem to always be aware and interested in me as a
person and not just as a therapist, they can sense if I am tired or pre-occupied and
immediately show concern and care, and this humbles me immensely and I feel so
very touched by them. Another sign of resilience is the refugees' sense of humour
and how we can sometimes laugh together about misunderstandings they tell me
about when they are dealing with various authorities.

Papadopoulos (2006) compares resilience and Adversity-Activated Development (AAD). He explains that the key characteristics of resilience are that the
refugee retains qualities that existed before, whereas AAD introduces new characteristics that did not exist before the adversity; in other words, refugees can be

strengthened by their particular exposure to adversity. We are social beings, and we are therefore always affected by others around us. According to Papadopoulos (2007), wider community ideology or views often affect refugees in more direct ways. Wider community and cultural contexts are active in forming at least part of the meaning systems of each individual.

Blackburn's (2010) theory is that people who have had adverse experiences often need assistance in finding ways to recover their lives from the effects of trauma and to build new lives which fit with their preferred sense of themselves. To me, this implies (and I have often seen it in my work with refugees) that they have the capacity and resilience within them and that they can access those inner strengths with help from the smaller and wider community, professionals and other networks. In this I agree with Melzak (1992) when she says that somehow, despite families being exposed to organised violence, torture and exile, some are able to build on their innate strengths, can hold on to ideas and beliefs and use the support of their networks. According to Melzak (1992), these families can use the natural healing processes of bereavement, dreams and play to work through difficulties. I agree with Rutter (1985) when he concludes that many people are not passive victims of organised violence but are able to become actively involved in changing their situation.

There is an increasingly held view that becoming a refugee is a purposeful act of strength and capability (Muecke, 1992; Ahern, 2000), and even though there is evidence that a minority of refugees are deeply troubled and need psychiatric intervention, the vast majority do not appear to be as psychologically dishevelled as one would expect, given the nature of some of their experiences. I agree with Alcock (2003) that powerful internal defences against intolerable loss and inner pain are mobilised within us to help us survive; however, I think they do not just help us survive but can be a driver for us to achieve more than just survival. This is already the case for some of my participants and patients, but I believe that with the right help and support, my other participants and patients who are still feeling more vulnerable, can also go beyond a state of survival to living more fully.

Effects of Trauma on the Individual

So much has been written on the effects of trauma on individuals, and it is a very important aspect of a refugee's reality. The amount of trauma refugees often survive is evident throughout my work with them; I am constantly reminded of the difficult experiences they have lived through before getting to the UK and once they arrive here. Even though I have spoken about some of the positive aspects of experiencing adversity, I also regard it as essential to allow space for my participants to share the pain and suffering they experience.

Alcock (2003) writes that the price of survival can aggravate loss of inner meaning and feelings of depletion and emptiness. People can be caught up in a cycle of repetition that makes it difficult to recover from these losses and to re-establish a life that has vivacity, purpose and meaning. She believes that the effects of acute losses and the impact of trauma do not disappear, although it is possible to regain a sense of hope and meaning in life. Alcock (2003) goes on to say that when home is lost, it is lost forever and even if we do go home, both home and we, ourselves, have changed. I often hear this with the refugees I work with where they describe feeling alienated in their home country and when reunited with family and friends left back home, as well as continuing to feel like an outsider in England; they seem to be left in a no-man's land where they are isolated and silent.

According to Varvin (1998), trauma puts the subject in a position in which he will re-experience not only the helplessness he felt as a child but also the strength and caring received. Varvin (2003) confirms that the effects of trauma are often long-lasting as the traumatic event forces its way into the individual, smashing through whatever barriers the mind has set up as a line of defence. This results in the loss of internal protection related to the internal other—primarily the loss of feelings of basic trust. When this internal linking is broken, damaged or destroyed, attachment to others may be perceived as dangerous. Withdrawal patterns may thus be the consequence, creating a negative spiral since withdrawal at the same time means the loss of potential support. When I think about my participants, I notice that none of them were in a state of withdrawal from professionals; on the contrary, they each seemed still hopeful about getting the right help.

Lewis (2012) writes that survivors of humanly designed traumas, the consequence of wars, imprisonment and torture, become ill from remembrances of their traumatic injuries, aspects of which return at night in ceaseless dreams and are re-lived by day in flashbacks and unbidden, intrusive memories. So tormented are these individuals by their repetitive reminiscences, that in treatment they frequently request help in forgetting. All the refugees I work with express this same dilemma and the wish and need to 'forget' their past harrowing experiences which haunt them on a daily basis. It is rather paradoxical because on the one hand they want to forget and on the other hand it is, to my mind, only through an accessible other mind that one can 'digest' the past traumas, by talking about the past and having a professional bear witness to one's adverse experiences.

Freud (1920) described trauma as the mind being pierced and wounded by events. He argued that

> an external trauma is bound to provoke a disturbance on a large scale in the functioning of the organism's energy and to set in motion every possible defensive measure. . . . When reality is unmanageable the defence must be equally extreme. The mind is flooded with stimulation, which cannot be borne, and to survive people must resort to defences that to others seem to be signs of madness.
>
> (1920: 607)

Moving to other psychoanalytical views, Winnicott (1971) describes trauma as an interruption to the sense of going on being, a fracture in the sense of continuity of the self. Garland (1998) concurs and refers to traumatic experiences as a break or rupture in one's sense of being. Winnicott (1971) and Garland's (1998) theorisation is consistent with my clinical experience of patients diagnosed with psychosis; dissociating or getting out of their bodies in order not to experience pain has become their way to survive trauma. The defences to which refugees resort in order to survive, stay on even after they are 'safe' in England and the coping strategy which has thus far helped them to survive now hinders them from living in society. Their minds stay in 'alert mode', always being prepared for flight when they no longer need to be. They need time and reassurance to no longer feel the need to be in flight mode, and every little pressure in life puts them straight back into being re-traumatised; this can be having to go for an interview at the job centre where they, once again, have to justify why they cannot work at the moment because of their psychological damage (often not visible), or when they receive a letter from housing to say they have to move. Their psyche is often so fragile that these everyday setbacks actually put them in a state of being re-traumatised and feeling hopelessly broken.

Although many of the refugees I work with do suffer from extreme defences, none of my participants spoke about extreme defences, such as disassociating, during their interviews. This may be because I only interviewed them for a few hours, which is not enough time to explore these matters in depth, and it may also have been because they knew our contact was time limited and that they would not have space to process these thoughts and feelings fully.

According to Alcock (2003), although people resume their lives after traumatic experiences, the impact does not disappear; I disagree with this because it is unhelpful to assume irrevocable damage from trauma. I have seen many of my clients heal through doing Eye Movement desensitisation and reprocessing (EMDR) with me, at a very slow pace and usually after a full year of just engaging with them and bearing witness to their pain and to their past.

Another example of extreme defence against trauma is the documentation by Van Boemel and Rozee (1992) of the phenomenon of post-traumatic nonorganic blindness in a group of more than 100 Cambodian women refugees from the Pol Pot genocide. These women were referred to Van Boemel for ophthalmologic diagnosis when no organic cause for their blindness could be found; each of them had witnessed horrific atrocities and each then post-traumatically stopped being able to perceive what her eyes were registering neurologically. Here, trauma is being somatically expressed (as I often see in my work with refugees who have suffered trauma) as an expression of unbearable pain and violence. Somatic presentations have been found to be higher among some racial and ethnic minorities, including Latinos and Asians (Dansky et al., 1996).

Fortuna (2009) speaks about studies which have suggested that psychological responses to trauma, such as fear, numbing, arousal, intrusive memories and avoidance of things and places that are reminders of the traumatic event, tend to be present in individuals across race and ethnicity (Charney and Keane, 2007; Clear, Vincent, and Harris, 2006). However, social stressors are important for understanding illness presentation and for facilitating the engagement of clients in treatment. For example, experiences of everyday racism and discrimination may be among the client's most prominent psychosocial stressors, adding significantly to his or her psychological distress. I think this is an extremely important point because as therapists we may focus on the past traumas of the refugee and not consider the influences of the clients' present context and social situation. I have often seen how my clients have gone back to having the same feelings of despair, anxiety and hopelessness when they have been faced with the risk of becoming homeless or losing any notion of safety and consistency. Fortuna (2009) also reminds us that guilt and shame about leaving others behind or the added fear of disputed legal status and discrimination can all add anxiety and fear that interact with post-traumatic stress disorder (PTSD) symptoms and related cognitions.

Papadopoulos (2001) argues that each individual's ability to 'read life' is a product of the connection between the 'mosaic substratum' of identity and the 'tangible' elements of one's identity. The mosaic substratum (Papadopoulos, 1997) refers to the fact that we belong to a country, a certain cultural group and language group and are used to a certain milieu. The loss of this mosaic leaves the individual with an inexplicable gap and a sense of unreality. The ability to 'read life' is the predictability that we get used to in living our everyday lives; ordinarily we are aware of which situations are to be avoided and which are not, when and how to behave and so forth. According to Papadopoulos (2001), it is this confidence that refugees lose as a result of their many losses, disorientation and frozenness. This is very evident from my participant Akbar's interview, where he speaks about how lost he felt when he first went to Sweden and had to learn about the underground system or getting money out of a cash point. Similarly, when I worked in a Red Cross refugee camp in Sweden, many of the refugees who came were treated as children by the staff at the camp because they were so lost in the new society. The Swedish staff were not informed enough about the refugees' past identities and the experiences they had lived through and were rather clueless and naïve about why they were so lost and inexperienced in the Swedish society. The more they were treated with condescension, the more childlike the refugees became.

Although I have been speaking about refugees, I must include asylum seekers in the discussion because a big part of the trauma my participants experienced was when they were waiting for a response from the Home Office. Procter (2005) speaks about how the uncertainty of asylum seekers' existence and strongly held beliefs that it is unsafe to return to their country of origin has taken an enormous physical and psychological toll on some.

Many studies have shown that political violence exposure is associated with psychiatric disorders, especially PTSD, other anxiety disorders and depression (Eisenman et al., 2003; Jaycox et al., 2002; Martin-Baro, 1989; McCloskey et al., 1995; Rousseau and Drapeau, 2004; Sabin et al., 2003). Eisenman et al. (2003) also found that clients in primary care settings reporting exposure to political violence had greater chronic pain, impaired physical functioning and diminished health-related quality of life. Scott (2008) agrees that the consequences of extreme trauma may not be limited to an emotional disorder, but physical injuries may result in pain which in many cases becomes chronic; the pain serves to intensify the emotional distress. Many of the refugees and asylum seekers I work with are only able to speak about their aches and pains rather than their past experiences before trust is established, and it is extremely important to move at their pace and to just listen and empathise with them and be curious about their somatic symptoms to help them feel listened to, cared for and contained. Only then can one begin to explore the reasons behind their pains and their past adverse experiences and losses.

Scott (2008) also asserts that PTSD is only one of many disorders that you might suffer from following an extreme trauma. Other common problems, he says, are phobia, depression, panic disorder and alcohol abuse or dependence. In my work with refugees, I have often seen how refugees use alcohol or drugs to numb their feelings and to help them sleep, but unfortunately, I have also seen how the alcohol can lead to violence, as James (2010) describes. In my interviews I did not ask about any dependencies, as there is often a sense of shame linked to the consumption of alcohol, and I believe that in order to have such a conversation, you would need to, over time, build trust in the therapeutic relationship. Indeed, the refugees I work with only divulge their use of alcohol and drugs after I have built a trusting relationship, which often takes months.

Woodcock (2001) implies that memories of violence can be so threatening to the psychological and physical integrity of the survivor that recollections are literally split off from consciousness. The psychoanalysts Laub and Auerhahn (1993) identify six levels of 'knowing psychic trauma', by which they mean the way in which memory and experience are internalised physically and psychologically. They suggest that atrocity may be processed at different levels by survivors and that the shattering manner in which torture and atrocity violate the physical and psychological boundaries of survivors frequently causes their recall of events to emerge in ways that may be fragmentary and disconnected. The first of these six categories of remembering which Laub and Auerhahn elaborate on is 'not knowing', where trauma is lost to memory by de-realisation, splitting and depersonalisation. There is therefore a conflict in which there is a wish to remember as well as an equally strong aversion to memories as they emerge. Second, survivors may experience 'fugue states', where they re-experience atrocity as vivid flashbacks in which their consciousness of being in the present is eliminated. Third, the survivor may experience 'fragments', where partial sensations of the experience of atrocity float in and out of consciousness without any obvious context. They may present as paranoid ideations. The fourth category which Laub and Auerhah describe is when survivors experience 'transference phenomenon'. Here, fragments of their traumatic experiences are grafted onto inner representations of themselves or others. This may translate, for example, in the therapist being experienced as clumsy or invasive. Fifth, survivors may experience 'overpowering narratives', where they believe that they have overcome their experiences of atrocity. Memories of extreme events can therefore be discussed in a detached manner without any feelings about what happened. However, their everyday lives may be filled with recollections, and they may have horrifying nightmares. Finally, survivors are often driven by 'life themes', where an organising principle connected to the experience of atrocity pre-dominates life choices that are made in the wake of the atrocity. This reminds me of a refugee family I worked with who had waited for their leave to remain for five years; their teenage daughter said she was going to be a lawyer to make sure other refugee families did not have to go through the same horrific experiences her family went through to be heard by the system in England.

Because the expression of PTSD can vary, the question has been raised as to whether the symptom criteria for the diagnosis of PTSD are biased towards traditional Western expressions of distress and are not applicable cross-culturally (Cervantes et al., 1989; Marsella et al., 1996). Even with the current *Diagnostic and Statistical Manual of Mental Disorders* (4th ed.; *DSM—IV*; American Psychiatric Association, 1994) criteria for the diagnosis of PTSD, the disorder has often been noted to have a very heterogeneous presentation, as evident in attempts to develop additional diagnoses that capture complicated presentations, such as complex PTSD (Briere, 1987; Resick and Miller, 2009). However, I agree with Fortuna (2009) when she emphasises that when treating clients from diverse cultures there is also a necessity to be sensitive to how their language and conceptualisation of illness or distress may reflect post-traumatic symptoms in addition to classic symptoms that define PTSD.

Afuape (2011) asserts that the diagnosis of PTSD contradicts the notion that it is normal to react severely to extreme events and suggests the existence of a cut-off point whereby distress changes from being a natural response to being a pathological response. She says that the symptoms can be viewed as adaptive responses to oppressive and abusive experiences. Although I strongly agree with Afuape, I would mostly say that a person suffers from PTSD if he/she/they still have insomnia, memory difficulties, withdrawal, fright and so forth when he/she/they are living in a safe environment and no longer need those lifesaving responses.

Watters (2001) discusses further criticisms of the use of the PTSD concept in non-Western cultures. The focus on the past trauma events as determining the current psychological difficulties may undermine the importance of the current situation and the ongoing stressors faced by the refugee. To me, one must look at the refugee's situation on multiple levels because the refugee often suffers from traumatic experiences of the past but also from his/her/their current situation of often social exclusion, isolation, unemployment, poverty and dependence and changed status within the family and the society.

Effects of Trauma on Family Relationships

Looking back on all the research which has been done to explore the effects of forced migration on the individual, we can begin to understand the complexities with which refugee families have to deal. Some of the refugee's experiences may have a more positive effect, such as helping the person change their view on life, become stronger and gain ambitions. However, others will have a more destructive effect. In my own experience of working with refugee families, I have seen how the adverse experiences have led to violence and disconnection within families; in my research, I was surprised to see the silence which reigned in the families of my participants.

I shall analyse the meanings of silence later in the book, but what I could see from the couples I interviewed was that the silence clearly broke the family bonds and distanced not only the couple from each other but also the children from their parents. Because I did not interview the children, my analysis is based on parents' accounts of isolating themselves from their children. They said how they have little patience, can get easily distracted by a flashback in the middle of a game with their child and how they often just wanted to be alone. The children in all these families have suffered atrocities at a young age and have equally lived the experience of being unable to count on their parents to keep them safe. They had to run away and face their fear of human cruelty. Their brains have therefore had to invest more in survival rather than in being able to invest in their learning and thinking brain; fear restricts, and safety allows and encourages learning and development (Treisman, 2017). Thorup et al. (2020) discuss how the parents' trauma can negatively affect the child's attachment patterns to his/her/their caregiver.

Once in England, children are confronted with parents who are depleted and have lost their identity as well as feeling isolated and unable to build relationships outside of the family. This is often because the atmosphere in their home is not one which allows the child to bring home friends and because parents are suspicious of 'others' and may at times warn children against building friendships; the new culture and society can be seen as hostile, and the parents' sense of being persecuted continues. The silence which often reigns in the families hinders children from expressing their thoughts and emotions. Often children are protective of their parents and do not want to cause them any more worries; they therefore suffer in silence. Furthermore, the loss of identity and change in the status of parents in the new society is confusing for children; Gaulejac (1987) speaks about children suffering from a neurosis of class where they cannot recognise themselves in the place and class the family holds in society, often compared to the position they held in their own country. I have seen this many times in my work where children seem to hold on to the past identity of their parents (in the home country) and thereby find it difficult to truly adapt to their new and different lives in the host country. This second generation will try to explain to their new friends that they come from a specific background where they lived a privileged life in their home country, and they are often met with either disbelief or disinterest from their peers.

Woodcock (2000) states that when extreme events ruin a parent's internal representations of their own parental attachments, they may in turn be incapacitated from offering good enough parenting to their children. However, the child's healthy impulses towards development mean that the parent is challenged to respond to their needs for involvement. Woodcock adds that sometimes the parent is unable to react, and the child then experiences a parent who is absent and is therefore very different to their former self. This was evident from my interviews with the couples, presented in the next chapter, who all described themselves as not being able to be present mentally and emotionally for their child. The need to isolate themselves was so strong for these participants that they had to prioritise their own needs over their child's at times. This is a phenomenon which I see all too often in my work with refugee and asylum-seeking families.

Melzak (1992) also suggests that children whose parents have been affected by their experiences of trauma may experience their parents as unavailable or absent emotionally even when physically present. In my experience, children tend to always blame themselves for the shortcomings of their parents, and young children may feel that they are the cause of their parents' withdrawal as a result of their own angry thoughts or actions. Refugee children, who can be separated from their parents and sent to different camps, for example, may believe that separation from their families is in some way their own fault, or they may wonder why their parents did not love them enough to prevent pain and separation.

Melzak (1992) goes on to say that refugee children may have a disharmonious development, where they have been forced towards independence in certain areas of their functioning, while in other areas they may be stuck or regressed. According to Melzak, if the adult to whom the child is attached is unavailable, physically or emotionally, then the child can feel neglected and overwhelmed. Lewis (2012) asserts that extreme situations destroy the capacity of language to convey meaning and destroy the sense of self of the victim, especially in relation to others.

According to Papadopoulos (2001), when families are forced to migrate, relationships undergo fundamental transformations, and role reversals are not uncommon. For example, as children usually assimilate faster than their parents, they get new responsibilities; mothers tend to attain new authority due to their involvement with their children at school and in the community, whilst fathers seem to become more isolated as they lose their traditional position—they become more vulnerable, especially without the authority of the work status they had in their home country (Papadopoulos, 1999a; Papadopoulos and Hildebrand, 1997). According to Burck (2005), research findings indicate that there are significant issues in family relationships when children learn the new language faster than their parents when families migrate (Burck, 1997; Lau, 1984; Papadopoulos and Hildebrand, 1997; Raval, 1996). Darvishpour (1999) sees the changed power balance in Iranian families in favour of women. I have also witnessed this in my work with Iranian families who had migrated to Sweden and in my work with Iranian families in England. It is customary in Iran that in the case of divorce the children are placed in their father's care; if the father is deceased, they are put in the paternal family's care. This is to ensure financial security for the child, as historically men provided for the family financially. Thus many women who were unhappy in their marital lives could not consider separating from their husbands. However, when they migrated to countries such as Sweden and England, where they learned that they have equal rights, they filed for divorce and often applied to have the children live with them. Bearing in mind that family members may suffer from PTSD, Lipton (1994) asserts that family members, who live with an affected person, tend to develop similar symptoms that accelerate marital discord. I have witnessed how the children, and often the wives, of patients who suffered from PTSD could show signs of being in 'alert mode' all the time, having nightmares, sleeplessness, depression and anxiety, as the reactions of, for example, the father/ husband were unpredictable and could be violent. In many cases I have worked with, where the father in the family suffered from severe PTSD, I had to inform the mother and children about how to keep safe and give their father space if he seemed overly irritated or on edge; I would often tell the woman to not wake the husband up from a deep sleep, for example, and to stay away as much as possible when he started to drink in the evening to help him sleep. I would tell the men to sleep in a separate room because many of them would suffer from horrendous nightmares and would inadvertently hurt their spouse if she was in the same bed. Addressing safety measures in these situations is essential, and the dangers and violence need to be voiced and explained as part of the therapy. Often these issues needed to be spoken about individually, as the husband did not want to lose face in front of his spouse and the wife was too cautious to speak freely in front of her husband; once trust was established, these serious concerns could be spoken about in the couple sessions, and even with the children.

Njie-Carr et al. (2020) discuss the importance of the woman's acculturation in the host society and how this can strengthen her to become more independent and to seek help when needed.

Scott (2008) describes people with PTSD as living in a bubble where others are regarded as not part of the same story. He goes on to say that because trauma affects people in becoming unusually irritable and emotionally numb and therefore unable to have warm feelings towards those closest to them, family relationships soon deteriorate. I agree with Scott that there is an understandable logic in estrangement from others if the trauma suffered is interpersonal, such as oppression, assault, or torture. A large part of my work with traumatised refugees is to create a space where they can slowly begin to feel safe. This can include asking them where they would feel comfortable for me to sit and even the tone of my voice, whether they feel more comfortable if I whisper, for example. I sit with them during long periods and just listen to them cry and repeat how difficult life is and how they have no hope, and I very gently let them know that I am there, bearing witness, not being overwhelmed, able to remain calm and contained, and when they finally look up, I have a warm and reassuring smile to greet them. With one patient who had been in prison in Iraq for ten years, we came to the end of the session and I could see she was not well and not ready to leave, so I stayed in the room with her and then she realised herself that our time was up, so she hastily left the room. I was worried for her, and my next patient was late, so I went outside to look for her and saw her huddled, almost in the foetal position, by the stairs of our building. I went to her very gently, calmly warning her that it was me and that I was going to gently touch her back, almost to bring her back to the present. As

I sat down next to her, she turned towards me and just broke down in tears in my arms. I sat there, stroking her hair, comforting her, telling her things would be better and that she was safe now, far away from the horrors of her past. She was soon feeling better, looked up at me, and smiled and said she looked forward to our next session. This, to me, was her saying she could now trust me with her distress and anguish and her pain and know that I would be there for her, every step of the way. Even though the importance of having clear boundaries is often emphasised in a therapeutic relationship, I think it is not always appropriate or helpful when working with such despair. Each therapeutic situation is unique, and one needs to adapt the boundaries and rules to the needs of the client. In this case, as in many other cases, I do not hesitate to offer physical contact and support, but I know, for example, not to overstep the boundaries when working with male clients; in those cases I give them a great deal of empathy and comfort through my expressions and words only.

Earlier I spoke about how silence in refugee families can also cause their isolation and distancing from the community; Scott (2008) also suggests that a trauma victim's difficulties in connecting with others may not be confined to the inner circle of close friends and family, but often includes everyday social encounters with the development of social anxiety or phobia. He says that a common consequence of extreme trauma is that the affected individual stops investing time and energy in others. Relationships are viewed as pointless and irritating, resulting in increasing isolation. The tolerance of friends and family is difficult; they may react by distancing themselves, thereby increasing the victim's sense of isolation still further. According to Scott, avoidance of others is as much a hallmark of posttraumatic stress as avoidance of reminders of the trauma. In the small research I have done and in my work with refugees, I have never had the sense that my participants or patients had stopped investing time and energy in their relationships with others because they viewed them as pointless, but rather that they did not have the energy and psychological strength to invest in anyone or anything. They seemed to need time to just isolate themselves, and perhaps to mourn the past and who they were individually and as a family. They needed time to 'find' themselves again in order to be able to 'be' with others around them. This need for isolation has large consequences for the family interactions where each of the parents has to almost hibernate to heal, leaving children to deal with changes and loss by themselves. Furthermore, children are almost forced into isolation because of their parents' mental state, and thereby the members of the family mutually influence each other to be pulled down into a negative cycle.

The development of uncharacteristic irritability is a common consequence of extreme trauma and is one of the diagnostic symptoms for PTSD in the *DSM-IV-TR* (American Psychiatric Association, 2000). Such anger can have very negative effects on relationships in a family, and considering the families in my research, where members have suffered trauma, one can imagine the levels of tension in the household where each member isolates himself/herself/themselves possibly to protect themselves and others from their anger and impulsive reactions. Scott

(2008) explains that as they are faced with this level of threat, there is a desire to totally control everything; when things do not run according to plan, they lose control and there is extreme anger over minor stresses. When I think of all the complications and difficulties with which refugee families are faced on a daily basis, there are few minor stresses, but rather things like threat of homelessness, racism, work discrimination, isolation and so forth.

If I think back to what Varvin (2003) says about traumatised people becoming withdrawn and unable to trust others, we can see how this can impact relationships in a family. In the couple relationships of my participants, as well as with the families I work with, I can clearly see a lack of trust in the other because they had each felt so vulnerable and helpless, unable to help the other. According to Varvin, the trauma allows the emotions of anxiety, aggression and depression to dominate and the meeting with the other person therefore becomes potentially frightening and may be felt as complicated and confusing. Varvin asserts that empathy is reduced to egocentricity, intimacy is seen as intrusion or exploitation, and care is turned to neglect. The community feeling may be abandoned and transformed into psycho-physiological dis-ease. One is no longer a part of a group and may experience a loss of the aspect of personal identity related to the group or the family. Developmentally this relates to the establishment of a sense of 'us'. In societies where the family and the group are the most important organising units of society, and where belonging to such a group is of fundamental importance for both personal and social identity, disturbances in this dimension may have grave disorganising effects.

Voulgaridou, Papadopoulos and Tomaras (2006) have written about the different challenges refugee families face in the host country, such as gender roles changing and 'oppositional discourses' (Papadopoulos and Hildebrand, 1997). Considering these experiences in combination with the silence I have come upon in my interviews, I can imagine how overwhelming it must feel for the family members. There seems to be so much to deal with, the traumas of the past and its effects, the difficulties of the present and trying to fit in to the society without losing one's roots and identity and the fear of the future in a foreign culture.

Ahlberg (2007) writes that in violent situations and oppression, the individual is deprived of making choices on how to belong; 'like a staged psychotic fantasy, the performances of the torturers enhance regression and activate extreme protective mechanisms and persecutor primary objects' (p. 57). According to Ahlberg (2007), it therefore becomes very difficult to preserve the memory of caring and protecting others in the subject's internal world, and thus to integrate what is happening and to give it any meaning. Laub and Auerhahn (1993) also depict trauma as disrupting the link between self and the empathic other; the victim's protective shield is somehow punctuated from the outside, resulting in a profound ego split which causes relationships to be compromised or invaded by chronically ambivalent behaviour. Ahlberg (2007) also writes about how trauma breaks the basic trust between humans and disrupts close bonds; it causes mutual blame or mistrust and creates barriers to intimacy. I believe therefore that the number one priority in therapy with traumatised refugees is to help build trust in the therapeutic relationship. This will, in turn, help the client to begin to build other trusting relationships.

In summary, refugees and their families undergo a considerable amount of distress and suffer from emotional, psychological and societal difficulties. They are indeed like broken vases which need to be pieced together with a great deal of care and patience. The fact that they are asylum seekers and refugees is confirmation of the trauma they have already endured in their country and on the way to 'freedom'.

Once in the host country, the adverse experiences continue and thereby hinder the process of healing the past losses and trauma. My interviews show how my participants have tried to survive the difficulties of the past and to deal with the now by going into their shells and isolating themselves from their partner, and to an extent also from their children. The responsibility they feel as parents encourages them to be at least physically present for their child, but in their minds they seem to be re-living the nightmares of their past repeatedly. The silence in the families which I have become aware of seems to have various meanings and functions which can be positive; however, the effect of the silence is extremely negative, as it distances the family members and destroys the close family bonds which are such a significant part of the culture in Middle Eastern communities. There clearly is tension between the individual's coping mechanism to survive (such as silence and withdrawal) and the negative impact this same coping mechanism can have on family relationships, creating splits and fractures rather than togetherness.

In my work with refugees, I was always told how angry they felt, so I had assumed there would be a lot of conflict in the families; the silence I found was more difficult, in a sense, as conflict is a way of communicating, connecting and not giving up; conflict is dynamic and usually brings change. The couples I interviewed seemed to have mostly given up on their couple relationship and were focused on trying to get through the day. The mistrust between the couple and a sense of 'he/she/they cannot help me and will not bear to hear' seemed to have given them a feeling of helplessness, loneliness and despair. Added to this is the refugees' sense of shame, which then causes them to isolate themselves from others in their smaller community as well as in society. The children grow up in an atmosphere of fear (of the past, present and future) and vulnerability and do not have parents on whom they can count to take charge and to make them feel safe and secure. Some children may build on their resilience when faced with these difficulties, but others will grow up feeling insecure and unheard and learning not to voice their feelings and thoughts. The effects of trauma can thus be carried through generations if help is not given in time and in an effective manner. If trauma is not transformed, it will most definitely be transferred.

References

Afuape, T. (2011), *Power, Resistance and Liberations in Therapy with Survivors of Trauma, to Have Our Hearts Broken*. London: Routledge Publications.

Ager, A. & Strang, A. (2004), *Indicators of Integration, Final Report*. London: Home Office.

Ager, A. & Strang, A. (2008), Understanding Integration: A Conceptual Framework. *Journal of Refugee Studies*, 21(2): 166–191.

Ahern, F.L. (ed.) (2000), *Psychosocial Wellness of Refugees: Issues of Qualitative and Quantitative Research*. New York: Beghahn Books.

Ahlberg, N. (2007), *'No Five Fingers Are Alike' What Exiled Kurdish Women in Therapy Told Me*. London: Karnac Books Ltd.

Alayarian, Aida. (2007), Trauma, Resilience and Creativity. In *Resilience, Suffering and Creativity*. London: KarnacBooks Ltd.

Alcock, M. (2003), Refugee Trauma: The Assault on Meaning. *Psychodynamic Practice*, 9(3): 291–306.

Atfield, G., Brahnbhatt, K. & O'Toole, K.K. (2007), *Refugees' Experiences of Integration*. Birmingham: Refugee Council and University of Birmingham.

Baasher, T.A. (2001), Islam and Mental Health. *East Mediterranean Health Journal*, 7: 372–376.

Bhui, K. King, M., Dein, S. & O'Connor, W. (April 2008), Ethnicity and Religious Coping with Mental Distress. *Journal of Mental Health*, 17(2).

Birkett, Diana. (July 2006), Cultural Dynamics in Counselling Refugees. *Healthcare Counselling & Psychotherapy Journal*, 6(3): 18–21, 4.

Blackburn, P.J. (2010), Creating Space for Preferred Identities: Narrative Practice Conversations about Gender and Culture in the Context of Trauma. *Journal of Family Therapy*, 32: 4–26.

Blackwell, R.D. & Melzak, S. (2000), *Far from the Battle But Still at War: Troubled Refugee Children in School*. London: The Child Psychotherapy Trust.

Briere, J. (1987), Post Sexual Abuse Trauma, Data and Implications for Clinical Practice. *Journal of Interpersonal Violence*, 2(4).

Burck, C. (1997), Language and Narrative: Learning from Bilingualism. In R.K. Papadopoulos and J. Byng-Hall (eds.), *Multiple Voices: Narrative in Systemic Family Therapy*. London: Duckworth.

Burck, C. (2005), *Multilingual Living, Exploration of Language and Subjectivity*. London: Palgrave Macmillan Publishers.

Cantle, T. (2005), *Community Cohesion: A New Framework for Race Diversity*. Basingstoke: Palgrave Macmillan.

Castles, S., Korac, M., Vasta, E. & Vertovec, S. (2002), *Integration: Mapping the Field*. London: Home Office.

Cervantes, R.C., Salgo de Snyder, V.N. & Padilla, A.M., (1989), Post Traumatic Stress in Immigrants from Central America and Mexico. *Psychiatric Services*, 40(6).

Charney M.E. & Keane, T.M. (April 2007), Psychometric Analyses of the Clinician-Administered PTSD Scale (CAPS)—Bosnian Translation. *Culture Divers Ethnic Minor Psychol*, 13(2): 161–168.

Cinnirella, M. & Loewenthal, K.M. (1999). Religious and Ethnic Group Influences on Beliefs and Mental Illness: A Qualitative Interview Study. *British Journal of Medicine and Psychology*, 72: 505–524.

Clear, P.J, Vincent, P. & Harris, G.E. (2006), Ethnic Differences IN Symptom Presentation of Sexually Abused Girls. *Journal of Child Sexual Abuse*, 15(3).

Crossley, D. (1995), Religious Experience within Mental Illness. Opening the Door on Research. *The British Journal of Psyhciatry*, 166: 284–286.

Dansky, B.S., Brady, K.T., Saladin, M.E., Killeen, T., Becker & Roitzsch, J. (1996), Victimization and PTSD in Individuals with Substance Use Disorders: Gender and Racial Differences. *The American Journal of Drug and Alcohol Abuse*, 22(1).

Darvishpour, M. (1994), Divorce among Iranian Immigrants. *The Iran Times.*

Darvishpour, M. (1999), Intensified Gender Conflicts within Iranian Families in Sweden. *Nora: Nordic Journal of Women Studies,* 7(11).

Dein, S. (2004), Working with Patients with Religious Beliefs. *Advances in Psychiatric Treatment,* 10: 287–294.

Eisenman, D.P., Gelberg, L., Liu, H. & Shapiro, Martin F. (2003), Mental Health and Health-Related Quality of Life among Adult Latino Primary Care Patients Living in the United States With Previous Exposure to Political Violence. *The Journal of American Medical Association,* 290(5).

Esmail, A. (1996), Islamic Communities and Mental Health. In D. Bhugra (ed.), *Psychiatry and Religion.* London: Routledge.

Fortuna, L.R. (June 2009), Minority and Refugee Clients. In K.T. Mueser, S.D. Rosenberg and H.J. Rosenberg (eds.), *Treatment of Posttraumatic Stress Disorder in Special Populations: A Cognitive Restructuring Program.* Washington, DC: American Psychological Association Press.

Freud, S. (1920), Beyond the Pleasure Principle. In Peter Gay (ed.), *The Freud Reader.* London: Vintage, 1989.

Garland, C. (1998), *Understanding Trauma.* London: Karnac Books.

Gaulejac, V. (1987), La névrose de classe: trajectoire sociale et conflits d'identité. In *Sociologie du travail,* 31e année n°2, Avril-juin 1989. Les comparaisons internationales. Théories et méthodes. Paris, France, pp. 267–268.

James, K. (2010), Domestic Violence within Refugee Families: Intersecting Patriarchal Culture and the Refugee Experience. *The Australian and New Zealand Journal of Family Therapy,* 31.

Jaycox, L.H., Stein, B.D., Kataoka, S.H., Wong, M., Fink, A., Escudero, O. & Zaragoza, C. (2002), Violence Exposure, Posttraumatic Stress Disorder, and Depressive Symptoms Among Recent Immigrant Schoolchildren. *Journal of the American Academy of Child and Adolescent Psychiatry,* 41(9).

Jenkins, A. (2011), Becoming Resilient: Overturning Common Sense—Part 1. *The Australian and New Zealand Journal of Family Therapy,* 32(1).

Knudsen, J. (1990), Cognitive Models in Life Histories. *Anthropological Quarterly,* 63(3): 122–133.

Knudsen, J. (1993), *Boat People in Transit: Vietnamese in Refugee Camps in the Philippines, Hong Kong, Japan.* Bergen: Department of Social Anthropology, dissertation.

Kohli, R. (2009), Understanding Silences and Secrets Whe Working with Unaccompanied Asylum-Seeking Children. In N. Thomas (ed.), *Children, Politics and Communication.* Bristol, England: Policy Press.

Lau, A. (1984), Gender, Power and Relationships: Ethno-Cultural and Religious Issues. In C. Burck and G. Daniel (eds.), *Gender, Power and Relationships.* London: Routledge, 1995.

Laub, D. & Auerhahn, N.C. (1993), Knowing and Not Knowing Massive Psychic Trauma: Forms of Traumatic Memory. *International Journal of Psychoanalysis,* 74: 287–302.

Lewis, J.D. (2012), Towards a Unified Theory of Trauma and Its Consequences. *International Journal of Applied Psychoanalytic Studies,* 9(4): 298–317.

Lipton, M.I. (1994), *Post-Traumatic Stress Disorder- Additional Perspectives.* Springfield, IL: CC Thomas.

Losi, N. & Strang, A. (2008), IntegraRef: Local Communities and Refugees, Fostering Social Integration. *Final Report.* Available at: www.evasp.eu/attachments/039-035-integraRef%20finalReport.pdf

Marsella, A.J., Friedman, M.J., Gerrity, E.T. & Scurfield, R.M. (1996), *Ethnocultural Aspects of PTSD: Some Closing Thoughts*. Washington, DC: American Psychological Association, xxii, pp. 576.

Martin-Baro, I. (1989), Political Violence and War as Causes of Psychological Trauma in El Salvador. *International Journal of Mental Health*, 18(1).

McCloskey, L.A, Locke, C.J, Southwick, K. & Fernández-Esquer, M.E. (1995), The Psychological and Medical Sequelae of War in Central American Refugee Mothers and Children. *JAMA Paediatrics*, 150(8).

Melzak, S. (1992), Secrecy Privacy, Repressive Regimes and Growing Up. *Bulletin of the Anna Freud Centre*, 15: 205–224.

Muecke, M.A. (1992), New Paradigms for Refugee Health Problems. *Social Science and Medicine*, 35(4): 515–523.

Njie-Carr, Veronica P.S., Sabri, Bushra, Messing, Jill T., Suarez, Cecilia, Ward-Lasher, Allison, Wachter, Karin, Marea, Christina X. & Campbell, Jacquelyn. (September 2020), Understanding Intimate Partner Violence among Immigrant and Refugee Women: A grounded Theory Analysis. *Journal of Aggression, Maltreatment & Trauma*.

Papadopoulos, R.K. (1999a), Working with Families of Bosnian Medical Evacuees: Therapeutic Dilemmas. *Clinical Child Psychology and Psychiatry*, 4(1): 107–120.

Papadopoulos, R.K. (1999b), Storied Community as Secure Base. *The British Journal of Psychotherapy*, 15: 322–332.

Papadopoulos, R.K. (April 2001), Refugees, Therapists and Trauma: Systemic Reflections. *Context*, 54.

Papadopoulos, R.K. (2002), *Therapeutic Care for Refugees: No Place Like Home*. London: Karnac Books.

Papadopoulos, R.K. (2006), *Refugees and Psychological Trauma: Psychosocial Perspectives*. London: Karnac Books.

Papadopoulos, R.K. (2007), Refugees, Trauma and Adversity-Activated Development. *European Journal of Psychotherapy and Counselling*, 9(3): 301–312.

Papadopoulos, R.K. & Hildebrand, J. (1997), Is Home Where the Heart Is? Narratives of Oppositional Discourses in Refugee Families. In R. Papadopoulos and J. Byng-Hall (eds.), *Multiple Voices: Narrative in systemic Family Psychotherapy*. London: Duckworth.

Procter, N.G. (2005), Providing Emergency Mental Health Care to Asylum Seekers at a Time When Claims for Permanent Protection Have Been Rejected. *International Journal of Mental Health Nursing*, 14: 2–6.

Raval, H. (1996), A Systemic Perspective on Working with Interpreters. *Journal of Child Psychology and Psychiatry*, 1: 29–43.

Resick, P.A. & Miller, M.W. (2009), Post Traumatic Stress Disorder: anxiety or Traumatic Stress Disorder. *Journal of Traumatic Stress*, 22(5).

Rousseau, C. & Drapeau, A. (2004), Premigration Exposure to Political Violence among Independent Immigrants and Its Association With Emotional Distress. *Journal of Nervous and Mental Disease*, 192(12).

Rutter, M. (1985), Resilience in the Face of Adversity—Protective Factors and Resistance to Psychiatric Disorder. *British Journal of Psychiatry*, 147: 598–611.

Sabin, M., Cardozo, B.L., Nackerud, L., Kaiser, R. & Varese. L. (2003), Factors Associated with Poor Mental Health Among Guatemalan Refugees Living in Mexico 20 Years After Civil Conflict. *JAMA*, 290(5).

Scott, M.J. (2008), *Moving on After Trauma: A Guide for Survivors, Family and Friends*. London: Routledge.

Smyth, G. & Kum, H. (2010), 'When They Don't Use It They Will Lose It': Professionals, De- Professionalization and Re-Professionalization: The Case of Refugee Teachers in Scotland. *Journal of Refugee Studies*, 23(4).

Spicer, N. (2008), Places of Exclusion and Inclusion: Asylum-Seeker and Refugee Experiences of Neighbourhoods in the UK. *Journal of Ethnic and Migration Studies*, 34(3). Taylor & Francis

Strang, A. & Ager, A. (2010), Refugee Integration: Emerging Trends and Remaining Agendas. *Journal of Refugee Studies*. 23(4). Oxford University Press.

Thorup Dalgaard, N., Høgh Thøgersen, M. & Riber, K. (2020), Transgenerational Trauma, Transmission in Refugee Families. The Role of Traumatic Suffering, Attachment Representations, and Parental Caregiving. In *Working with Refugee Families (Trauma and Exile in Family Relationships) Transgenerational Trauma Transmission in Refugee Families*. Volume 10.1017/97

Treisman, K. (2017), *Working with Relational and Developmental Trauma in Children and Adolescents*. London: Routledge.

Van Boemel, G.B. & Rozee, P.D. (1992), Treatment for Psychosomatic Blindness among Cambodian Refugee Women. *Women and Therapy*, 13(3).

Vangelisti, A.L. & Caughlin, J.P. (1997), Revealing Family Secrets: The Influence of Topic, Function and Relationships. *Journal of Social and Personal Relationships*, 14: 679–705.

Varvin, S. (2003), Extreme Traumatisation: Strategies for Mental Survival. *International Forum of Psychoanalysis*, 12(1): 5, 12.

Varvin, S. & Hauff, E. (1998), Psychoanalytically Oriented Psychotherapy with Torture Victims. In I. Jaranson and J.M. Popkin (eds.), *Caring for Victims of Torture*. Washington, DC: American Psychiatric Press, pp. 117–130

Voulgaridou, M.G., Papadopoulos, R.K. & Tomaras, V. (2006), Working with Refugee Families in Greece: Systemic Considerations. *Journal of Family Therapy*, 28: 200–220.

Vrecer, N. (2010), Living in Limbo: Integration of Forced Migrants from Bosnia and Herzegovina in Slovenia. *Journal of Refugee Studies*, 23(4): 484–502.

Wade, A. (March 1997), Small Acts of Living: Everyday Resistance to Violence and Other Forms of Oppression. *Contemporary Family Therapy*. Human Sciences Press Inc.

Watters, C. (2001). Emerging Paradigms in the Mental Health Care of Refugees. *Social Science and Medicine*, 52.

Watts, R.J., Griffith, D.M. & Abdul-Adil, J. (1999). Sociopolitical Development as an Antidote for Oppression: Theory and Action. *American Journal of Community Psychology*, 27(2): 255–272.

Winnicott, D. (1971), The Location of Cultural Experience. In *Playing and Reality*. Harmondsworth: Penguin Books, 1985.

Woodcock, J. (October 2000), A Systemic Approach to Trauma. *Context, The Magazine for Family Therapy and Systemic Practice*, 51: 2–4.

Woodcock, J. (2001), Threads from the Labyrinth: Therapy with Survivors of War and Political Oppression. *Journal of Family Therapy*, 23: 136–154.

Chapter 3

Refugees' Lived Experiences

This chapter is based on my interviews with two Afghani couples, one Iraqi couple and one Iranian couple. The couples were recruited through the NHS as well as voluntary organisations working with refugees. Although they were recruited as couples, I interviewed each person individually, at their request. I believe this enabled them to speak more freely about their feelings and thoughts and to recount their experiences, without having to take into consideration the impact on their partner or their relationship. I asked them about their lived experiences of trauma; in their country, during their journey to England and once they arrived in England and were waiting for their refugee status. After discussing their lived experiences, I went on to ask more about how these traumatic events have affected them as individuals and in their relationships with their partner and their children. The interviews with the Afghani couples and the Iranian couple were conducted without the help of an interpreter, as I speak Farsi. The interview with the Iraqi couple was done with the help of an interpreter with whom I had worked for many years as a CAMHS family therapist. Following my colleague Dr Asen's advice, I asked the interpreter to sit behind the participants so that they were facing me directly and there was less a feeling of intrusion; we felt more connected.

Each participant expressed how important it is for their voice to be heard, and they were extremely generous in sharing their thoughts and experiences with me without hesitation. They each expressed a wish for me not to contact them again after their interviews; they did not want to have the transcripts or have any sight of this book (although they had given permission for their interviews to be published). When I explored this further, each person explained that they wanted to use the opportunity of the interviews to 'empty' themselves of all the past pain and suffering and to know that they never needed to see me again. The interviews were an immensely emotional experience for me because I could only be a witness to their pain as a researcher, whereas when I work with refugees as a systemic therapist, as well as an Eye Movement desensitisation and reprocessing (EMDR) practitioner, I try to give help and support in various ways.

I would like to invite the reader to feel and understand the struggles of these families but also their sense of resilience and humanity. I shall present each of the

DOI: 10.4324/9781003310716-4

families by using quotes from their interviews to demonstrate their experiences in three phases: pre-flight, when they lived in their home country; flight, when they took the decision to leave everything behind and emigrate; and post-flight, when they arrived in the UK and applied for refugee status.

In working with refugees, I have come to notice how important it can be to repeat their story, in detail, over and over again. This was similar in these interviews because the quotes were repeated several times. I believe the need for repetition to be linked to the trauma experienced whereby the more the person repeats their adverse experiences the more this process helps them to 'digest' what they have lived through. There is also a sense of wanting to make sure they are heard and that this particular aspect of their experience is acknowledged; that someone is bearing witness to their pain and suffering.

Another phenomenon I have become aware of in working with refugees is a 'lost' or confused sense of time; refugees often speak in the present tense because their experiences are still very real in their minds, making them feel vulnerable and constantly at risk.

Pre-Flight

Refugees leave their home country because they have no choice; but they all have different experiences in their country. Some refugees leave because of their political activities and the repercussions on them and their families and the fear for their life. Mahdi and Fatemeh are from Iraq, and Mahdi comes from a family where they were all politically active, as was Mahdi. He was a known political activist, and he was therefore granted political asylum even before arriving in the UK. After living in England for two years he was able to get a visa for his wife, Fatemeh, and their ten-year-old son, Rooh. During the two years they were left in Iraq, Fatemeh had to flee from one town to the next together with Rooh and her mother-in-law, as they were being persecuted by the Iraqi Secret Service. During their marriage, Fatemeh and Mahdi were never allowed to live a quiet life because of Mahdi's activities against Saddam Hossein's regime, and both he and his family paid the price for this. Fatemeh is now pregnant with their second child.

Fatemeh spoke with great emotion about the level of persecution and surveillance the couple were under due to her husband's political activities. She recalls with a sense of despair how the Iraqi Secret service, Al Mokhabarat, would come for her husband:

They would come into my home looking for my husband . . . day and night. They used to take him off to prison. They came . . . twenty of them and took him away. . . . They banged on the door and came in, threw things all over the house . . . they were terrible; they would sometimes break the front door. For the twelve years we were married they would come into our home and take him away for interrogations.

Although her husband fled the country two years before she and her son could, Fatemeh continued to experience constant pressure and verbal and emotional abuse by the Iraqi regime; pressure to betray her husband:

> *They would come to take me for interrogations; they would ask me where my husband was, why he left, how he left. I was afraid they would kill us instead of him or imprison me to get him to come back . . . as they often do. They would barge into the house and interrogate me about my husband all the time.*

During these two years of surviving without her husband's presence, Fatemeh and Rooh experienced yet another level of oppression, they were forced to live a nomad's life in constant fear: '*We kept moving from city to city and house to house all the time so the intelligence services wouldn't find us and interrogate us again.*'

Mahdi also recounted the ordeals he lived through in his home country; he described a life of oppression and violence on behalf of the Iraqi Regime:

> *Every time we (me and my brothers) got arrested, we were not sure to come out alive and I couldn't risk hiding at people's homes I was not 100% sure of. Before I stayed with anyone, I would make sure their phones weren't hacked, etc. In Iraq every time I went out, I was afraid I would get arrested, tortured or killed.*

Mahdi was arrested in 2000 and was in prison for three months, and in 2002 he was arrested again and was imprisoned for 15 days:

> *every time under severe torture. Because of the torture, I am deaf in my left ear and paralysed in my right arm; not to talk about the mental torture. From the moment we got out of the car they transported us in, until we were released three months later, we were blindfolded. It was only during interrogations that they took off the blindfold, but the interrogator would stand behind you and they would hit from behind and you had no right to turn around. I made the mistake of turning around once, and they paid me a lesson which leaves me deaf to this day. I was always in isolation. We were always blindfolded otherwise, if we wanted to go to the loo, in the cell, always. It was very difficult times. During this process you would get beaten, given electric shocks and tortured in general. One time they had recorded what I thought was my son's voice and they played it to me; I thought my son was there and was extremely distressed. I did believe they had brought my son and wife, though, and at other times I thought 'no' but they had put doubt in me, which was torture in itself. I didn't really know anything anymore, you had no idea about the day, the night, the time and I knew they were capable of everything.*

Mahdi was mindful of the impact of his arrest on his wife: '*I was taken to prison, for ten days my wife had no news of me and didn't know where they had taken me or whether I was still alive.*'

Refugees have often suffered cruelty at the hands of their fellow countrymen in their country, and to me this is one of the most painful experiences because as human beings we have a sense that we should feel secure in our 'home' country and be understood and accepted, and when our human rights are violated by the country we were born in, it makes life unbearable. Mahdi described this sense of helplessness and the feelings of anger which go hand in hand with it:

> *I remember the judge had a beard and he treated us like animals. He didn't even look at us, he just asked his secretary if we were the 'x' brothers, and when she said yes, he said, 'I have given their sentence already, make sure it is executed'. We didn't know what our sentence was, but they blindfolded us and took us to prison. We didn't even know it was prison they were taking us to. We didn't even know we were being taken to Baghdad!*

A life in hiding usually means a life of secrets, mistrust and deceit. During her interview, Fatemeh repeatedly spoke about her ordeal of having to keep secrets from all her family members and close friends. Because Fatemeh's husband had fled the country and come to England, Fatemeh could not let anyone know that she knew where he was; she could not trust anyone enough to tell them: '*My husband kept warning me about telling people. I could not utter a word to anyone, I could not take the risk of trusting anyone with my thoughts.*' Even when Fatemeh and her son were leaving to join Mahdi in England, she had to pretend they were just visiting family in Baghdad with her son. She couldn't tell her son either because she could not trust him to keep the secret. This was extremely difficult for Fatemeh, as she could see how much her son worried about his father and she couldn't tell him she knew his father was safe. There are spies everywhere in Iraqi society, and Fatemeh could not take the risk of her son saying anything about his father in school.

Because Fatemeh couldn't tell her mother they were leaving Iraq for good, she never got to hold her mother in her arms and say goodbye:

> *It is very hard. A week after I had left, my parents called my mother-in-law, worried, because they had not heard from me and she told them I had gone to my husband. My mother could not understand how I could leave her without saying goodbye.*

Although resilience and resistance are not the same, I have seen how they often merge, as the inner resilience of the individual, couple and family as a whole is a form of resistance to the oppression they are/have been under.

Fatemeh had to live a life of resistance, as not only did she have to put up with enormous pressure from the government but also from her family, who wished for a more traditional, quiet married life for her. Fatemeh recounted how her brothers kept insisting she leave her husband:

> but I stood firm because I love him so much and that's what kept me going. I would of course deny this to the Al Mokhabarat and say that I had separated from him, that I had asked for a divorce.

For two years Fatemeh resisted the Al Mokhabarat and kept her husband's whereabouts secret, even though she was under constant pressure.

Mahdi recounted a life of resistance against the Iraqi Regime, but he also recalls being resilient in prison and thinking he would not let them break him:

> I was not afraid, but I was worried, worried for my family. I felt my life had come to an end the way they spoke, and I had accepted it; I was mentally prepared for prison. The Al Mokhabarat person saw I wasn't afraid and said: 'I am going to make sure you are executed, but not right away.' I said calmly: 'as you wish.' One time they had recorded what I thought was my son's voice and made me believe my son was in prison too. I was extremely distressed, but I did not show them my distress. The guard even said to me: 'you traitors are without any feeling, so cold.' After all the torture, they got no information out of me.

However, no matter how resilient one might be, being at the mercy of others brings feelings of helplessness and fear. Fatemeh spoke with great emotion about her feelings of helplessness and constant fear with regard to all the violence she and her son were subject to.

> They (Secret Service) didn't leave us a life to live. We had no life, no life. Rooh was so doubtful that we could get out of Iraq and kept asking: 'Is it possible? Can we really go?' My son was so terrified at the time, nervous all the time. He would be petrified and cry all the time. His father just disappeared, and he did not believe he would see him again. Rooh has seen me crying in despair and fear all of his life, moving our things in a hurry, always on guard and it has affected him, he was (is still) always frightened, he couldn't sleep and kept thinking his father was dead.

From the moment Mahdi was arrested, he was also helpless and vulnerable, at the mercy of others; 'We didn't know what our sentence was. All three of us (brothers) became very stressed and anxious because we knew that going to Baghdad meant most probably never coming back alive. Like so many others before us.'

Many refugee families I work with describe how their lives were turned upside down through circumstances such as being in the wrong place at the wrong time, getting on the wrong person's bad side (persons in power) and being in disbelief about the level of harassment they may be subjected to. While valuing Watts, Griffith and Abdul-Adil's (1999) description of oppression as the unjust use of power by one socially salient group over another in a way that creates and sustains inequality, I would add Gil's (1998) definition of injustice: 'coercively establishing and maintaining inequalities, discrimination, and dehumanising, development-inhibiting conditions of living . . . imposed by dominant social groups, classes, and people upon dominated and exploited groups, classes and peoples' (p. 10). Van Wormer (2004) argues that injustice refers to a general lack of rights or justice, whereas oppression refers to the mistreatment of people. However, for the purpose of this book I will not make a distinction between injustice and oppression, as I argue that injustice is oppressive.

Another couple who suffered persecution and severe injustice in their country is Tina and Hamed. Tina and Hamed lived a happy and prosperous life in Afghanistan. However, they lived in Taliban territory, and Hamed was suspected of political activity because of his friendship with intellectual and forward-thinking people.

Hamed owned a restaurant and in order to find out more information about Hamed's connection with intellectuals who were against the Taliban regime, a Taliban was placed in their restaurant to watch their every move. The Taliban gave information to one of their leaders, who changed their lives forever. The Taliban leader, or sheikh, became attracted to Tina and kidnapped and raped her, making her understand that he was expecting to have a relationship with her.

Tina never shared her ordeal with her husband. The family fled Afghanistan with the help of smugglers. These same smugglers made them travel for months between various countries in Europe under extremely difficult conditions. The family was finally forced to travel to England separately. Hamed came first; he was arrested at the airport and put in jail for six months.

Tina recounts:

From the day after my husband's arrest for interrogation, I saw this 50–60-year-old man, who obviously had a position in the Taliban, come to the restaurant. My husband said to me that he was a Taliban who was going to be spying on us.

Tina quickly began to feel vulnerable and uneasy around him:

I noticed he kept thinking of excuses to talk to me. I had already sensed he was looking at me all the time, but I was used to these dirty Taliban being like that. One time, I was alone and one of his bodyguards came and gave me a package. It was a new and very expensive mobile phone; I was shocked at his audacity because he could see I was a married woman; what was all this about? I felt a tremble in my stomach.

Tina soon realised that the Taliban knew all about her. He had investigated her, and she described how, a few days after he had tried to give her the present (which she had refused), she was taken away by two Taliban men under his orders.

That day as I was walking home, I felt a car was following me. I cannot explain that instant and what goes on inside of you then, I felt petrified. The car stopped next to me, and one of the men asked me to get into the car, as they wanted to ask me questions. When you've been living in such an oppressive atmosphere as in Afghanistan, you know you cannot question their orders, so even though I wanted to run away, I got into the car and started to ask them what they wanted, who they were, etc. Suddenly, the man on my left pushed my neck and head down in a way that I was bent down and couldn't move, and he said, 'you talk too much'. One of the Taliban hit me.

Tina thought she was being taken away to be interrogated about her husband's intellectual friends and their activities, but she soon realised the Taliban sheikh wanted her:

He came and sat next to me and said: 'one thing I have always wanted to know is the length of your hair.' As he took off my head scarf I trembled with fear. I had been expecting to be interrogated and this was something else. He said: 'Do you want me to take you away for a week? You deserve to have a holiday, you shouldn't work.'

However, as Tina resisted his advances, the Taliban became aggressive and violent:

He said to me 'look, if I want to, I can attach you to this radiator and do what I want to you, so don't waste your time resisting me. As he was saying these things to me, he was physically getting closer to me, and I was in the corner of the sofa. So in the end . . . I don't know . . . he did whatever he wanted to do to me. He did everything he felt like doing to me for a few hours. He raped me in every possible way he could.'

Tina did not speak of this to her husband and pretended like everything was okay, but she realised the Taliban was not finished with her.

I went to my husband's work the next day (after the rape) and saw the Taliban coming in!! He looked at me with a smile as if to say that we were familiar. I mean he looked at me as if he had won and gotten what he wanted. He said in a flirty voice: 'Your hijab is never really good is it?' As he said it, he adjusted my hijab and he touched me, and I realised he was going to touch me in public now and there was no stopping him from raping me again. I knew he was touching me as if to say, 'do you remember? I knew then that we had to run away.'

Tina's husband, Hamed, had been arrested for interrogation because of his association with friends who were intellectual and therefore against the Taliban. He recounted how the Taliban barged into his restaurant after he had gathered with his friends there. They arrested him in order that he would give his friends' names away.

A large part of Hamed's experience of trauma is related to his sister, with whom he had an extremely close relationship. Because Hamed and his wife and children had gone into hiding (after the Taliban had gotten involved in their lives), he had asked his sister to go to their flat to get some of his belongings and papers. She therefore became fully involved in the harassment they were victim to.

> She (sister) had gone to the flat and found the papers I had asked for and taken them. The Taliban had then followed her from the flat. They arrested her, and I cannot imagine what they did to her in the interrogation; every time I talk about it or think about it, I feel like I am dying. When they captured my sister, I realised it was time to leave Afghanistan because they would've found me and killed me otherwise. They interrogated her for several hours and during that time we were fleeing Afghanistan; they took her back for interrogations several times. This happened in December, and I know that they caught several of my intellectual friends in January and within ten days they were all executed.

To me it was clear that Hamed seemed to be more affected by the violence and cruelty his sister suffered 'because of him', rather than the violence he himself was a victim to. His feelings of guilt and self-blame were torturing him.

I have spoken about all the secrets Mahdi and Fatemeh had to live with and endure to stay alive. In Hamed and Tina's case the secrets became necessary to protect the couple. Tina never told her husband she had been taken away and raped. He therefore still believes the family were forced to leave Afghanistan because of him and his intellectual friends. Tina described how she had to keep everything to herself when she went home after having been raped.

> Now I had to think of an explanation for my children, I started to make up a story. I was thinking 'what shall I do? Shall I tell my husband? Shall I try to forget it? Shall I pretend it never happened?' If I told my husband I knew he would kill the Sheikh and then our whole life would be destroyed. I needed to talk to someone, but who and how?

To protect her family, Tina had to endure the ordeal she had been through in isolation and secrecy, putting up a smile for her family and entourage. She understood, however, that the sheikh had taken her silence as an invitation to continue to use her for his sexual pleasures whenever he wished to. They were sharing a secret which put her at constant risk. Tina had to convince her husband to leave.

Couples' Past Lives Before They Were Interrupted

An important part of the interviews seemed to become giving the interviewees an opportunity to speak about their past identities, stories, lives, who they were before all the trauma and hardships affected them so. As each spoke about their past, I could see a difference in their manner of speech, becoming more confident, their eyes becoming brighter, as if, for an instant, they were back to being that person, that couple, that family. It was only Mahdi and Fatemeh who did not speak of their past identities because Mahdi had always been politically active in Iraq and Fatemeh had always lived in fear of losing him throughout their married life.

Tina spoke with pride of her husband's success in Afghanistan and of her own ambitions before the Taliban took over.

He became a restaurant owner. He made it a very successful business, and we were happy. It was a big restaurant with five chefs and was situated on three floors. He provided everything for me, but I needed to be active in society, be around people. I wanted to be active, and I felt extremely oppressed at the idea of not being allowed to be active in society. When we were in Afghanistan, before the Taliban took over our territory, everyone at work used to say I was like a rainbow because every day I wore different things, different colours, and I used to go far to get to my hairdresser, who was the best in town, to make sure I always looked nice.

Tina spoke of her husband with warmth and care.

We had cultural differences, my husband and I, but we loved each other so much that these things were never a problem. We were always travelling in Afghanistan. My husband loved life and travelling and having fun. We had built our lives with love and care; everything in our flat was a result of months of searching, thinking. We had worked so hard to get to where we were; our life had become stable, comfortable, despite the Taliban, because in our home we were one with each other. My husband had friends, good friends, all over Afghanistan.

As Hamed remembered his past life in Afghanistan, his posture changed and he was sitting up straight, looking confident and full of energy. His voice was animated as he recounted his happy and successful past.

In Afghanistan we had a stable life; we had a status, went on holidays and lived a nice easy life where we both worked hard but also enjoyed life. Our whole life has changed here. Our house was like a hotel, so many guests, so much joy. We travelled so much, always going to new places. When I first bought the restaurant (my last one) it was going downhill, but I bought it knowing I could make a success out of it, and I did! I did! I paid off all the debts and started to make a profit; so much so that we bought another restaurant.

To me, this is why it is so important to allow the refugee to go back in time and to remember who they were and where they come from, so that they can feel that sense of self again; so that they can feel proud and hold their head up high. I do this in almost every one of my sessions with refugees to reinforce their inner identity, their inner resilience and a sense of respect for themselves; then they can begin to heal and adapt to a new way of life in exile.

I am touched and impressed by the level of courage and the sense of justice the refugees I work with show and have shown, in all the hardships; how they have still said 'no' at points where their lives were in danger. At other times, their resistance may have been more subtle, as Tina described in her interview; how when the Taliban sheikh gave her the present, she refused it, knowing she was putting herself at risk. When she was kidnapped by the sheikh's men, Tina recalled how her mind was racing as she was being driven to her dark destiny, with her head held down by force, all the time thinking she was going to be interrogated about her husband's friends.

> *I was thinking concentrate and think about the kind of answers you are going to give when they ask you questions about the intellectual friends; I kept thinking I wished I had asked my husband that night, when he came after being interrogated, what he had said, what he had heard so that I could say the same things. What shall I say to not put him [her husband] into trouble? I kept cursing myself for not having asked my husband these things to be prepared for a time like this.*

Then, when Tina realised with horror the real reason for her kidnapping, she persisted in resisting and pushed his hand away. In this nightmare, Tina continued to hold her children in mind and wished to live for them:

> *Until then I was sure he would kill me after (the rape), but when he said that he could give me a nice life I realised I would stay alive. I just wanted to get out alive, in whatever condition. I was happy to be alive and to be going home to my family.*

When she finally came home, Tina continued to show strength to protect her children from being harmed and knowing what their mother had lived through '*As soon as I got home from my ordeal, I changed the subject and asked the boys about their day, etc. I just went into my mother role; it was like a film playing in front of me.*'

Tina kept it together and even went into work the day after to not make her husband suspect anything was wrong, but when she saw the sheikh walk into the restaurant with a smile, her heart sank, and when he touched her without shame in public, as if to say he possessed her, she knew she had no choice but to resist him openly.

> *I felt like I wanted to kill him [the sheikh]. I exploded and pushed him back with great force. I don't know where I got the force from, but I insulted him in*

every way I could. My husband and the restaurant staff heard me screaming and shouting, and they came to help me. I hit him badly, I kicked him and punched him as I shouted at him.

Hamed recalled having heard his wife screaming and shouting:

I came upstairs and saw that my wife was in an argument with the Taliban sheikh and his men. He was being rude to my wife, and I therefore came to defend my wife and it became physical. The waiters came to our help because they knew the Taliban would have taken us to prison.

Having worked a lot with Afghani refugees, I asked whether he just thought they would have gone to prison or, worse, executed, and Hamed said for sure they would have been executed, as you cannot get away with attacking a Taliban sheikh. The restaurant staff helped them to get away from the restaurant, and the family went into hiding. Hamed needed to get some official papers from their flat, so he asked his sister to get them for him, not knowing whether the Taliban had already ransacked their home or not. He spoke with great emotion and pride about his sister and her courage when she went to their flat to get Hamed's papers for him. '*She realised she was being followed and had stopped at a crossing, at the red light, and before they realised, she jumped out of her car and had thrown all the papers in a river that flows by that road.*' As Hamed spoke about the river by the road in Afghanistan, I remember suddenly having childhood memories of Tehran. There are rivers alongside all the roads in Tehran as well, and the sound of the water running is very peaceful. I thought then that I would always see them differently now; I think I will always have Hamed's sister in mind, with fear in her stomach and braveness in her heart, protecting her brother by destroying his papers in the flowing water.

Despite showing great resilience, the feeling of helplessness was omnipresent in Tina's interview.

You don't have a choice but to go, as you know, Shadi. You cannot say no. You cannot object when you have been living in the atmosphere of oppression in Afghanistan. You just don't dare object, and you don't have the force either. I cried and wondered whether I would get out of that house alive. I had heard of so many people just disappearing, and I knew I would be one of them. The rape was like a nightmare, as if it hadn't happened to me; I still cannot believe what happened to me. I knew there was nothing I could do to stop the sheikh. I was powerless; when he touched me with his fingers, it just reminded me of how he had forced me to accept things and do things because I had no choice.

The family had no choice but to flee Afghanistan with the help of smugglers. This was the beginning of the next chapter in their struggle to stay safe and to keep their children from harm as much as they possibly could. I will return to this in the 'Flight' section.

Other Reasons to Leave Your Home Country

Some families leave their home country because they believe they can find a better or more prosperous life elsewhere; these are not necessarily economic refugees because they have a comfortable life financially in their home country, but they make the choice of leaving because they want their children to have a better education or they want to be able to advance more in their career. In Siavash and Pooneh's case they decided to leave Iran mostly because Siavash wanted to get away from his family. Siavash had lived in France for many years as a young student. When he went back to Iran, he was disappointed by his family and the Iranian society he found back home, finding them selfish and feeling alienated from their way of thinking. Pooneh was brought up in Iran and had a very successful practice as a nutritionist, a good social life and was generally happy.

When the couple got married, Siavash insisted they try to move away from Iran to start their life together without the interference of his family. The young couple decided not to tell their parents, knowing that they would disapprove. Their ordeal began when they decided to leave. I suppose, for this couple, the definition 'forced flight' is not appropriate because both Siavash and Pooneh chose to leave Iran for family reasons. However, speaking to Siavash, I realised he felt he had no choice because of his family and the people surrounding him, who were putting him down and treating him as a foreigner. I suppose in a way he tried to seek refuge outside of Iran for social reasons rather than political reasons. However, according to Siavash, he was forced to leave. They applied for a visa to France for Pooneh on three occasions and were refused each time; that is when they decided to leave and seek refuge in France. Due to their decision to leave Iran without telling their respective parents, the couple's life started with lies and secrets. Pooneh spoke about having lied to her family and not telling them they were going to seek 'refuge' in another country out of shame, as her family would not have understood her choice of becoming a refugee.

> We decided not to tell our families. If my father ever found out that I was going to do something like that, become a refugee, he would be furious at me. I didn't dare to tell my parents I was seeking asylum. I had to lie to my mom and said that I had finally gotten a visa for France and was going there.

Siavash, on the other hand, said that he had not decided to hide the truth from their families out of shame but out of mistrust.

> No one in our family or friends knew that we were leaving. We hadn't told anyone anything. We just told them we were going on vacation. I just didn't trust anyone. That's why I didn't tell anyone, and I still think it was the right

decision. My wife's parents knew we were not on holiday and that we would not be going back, but they did not know how we were going to Europe.

Pooneh recounted how from the beginning of their marriage they had discussed leaving Iran.

My husband had a permit to live in France because he had grown up there. He refused to leave Iran without me. We didn't want to stay in Iran because my husband could not fit in and make his life there, as he had been away from Iran for too long. He had come back to Iran but didn't have the same mentality as everyone else. He doesn't have the Iranian mentality you need to have when dealing with Iranians. We had just gotten married at the town hall but were still living separately because we had not had the marriage ceremony.

When Pooneh said this, I remember how she looked at me intensely to see if I understood what she meant, and I nodded with empathy; the couple had spent their first night as a married couple in a bed in refuge in an unknown country. They had run away together, and I shall describe their flight in the next part of this chapter. However, because their life together as a couple had started off with such difficulty, each of their past lives seemed to be even more important, especially for Pooneh:

I had been brought up in comfort, safety and love. I loved my house; I especially loved my bedroom. I had bought a beautiful chandelier for it and had decorated it so that I loved spending hours in my room. I also had a very successful practice as a nutritionist and had many patients. My husband was the nicest, sweetest guy, and I felt meeting him was the best thing that had happened to me. We were so very much in love. He used to adore me, and we used to love spending time together, talking for hours.

Siavash spoke about his life in Iran with great emotion and sadness.

I lived outside of Iran for many years and then decided to go back home when I finished my studies. I felt like a stranger and did not feel a part of the society in Iran anymore; I didn't fit in in either Europe or Iran, I was in between and a stranger to both. But I knew that in Europe I had felt happier and calmer because at least no one [family] was bothering me and giving me grief. At first, I wanted to go back to France where I had been brought up; I applied for a visa for my wife several times, but three times they refused, so we were obliged to leave Iran illegally. You know, unfortunately, the memory and idea I had of family relations in Iran did not turn out to be right. Things had changed, and there wasn't the closeness and loving relationships I had experienced before in the family and with friends. I felt distant to everyone; I couldn't trust anyone, and I had been betrayed over and over again in the five years I had lived in Iran after having gone back. I was getting so depressed in Iran, going nowhere, I had nothing left, and my dreams had been shattered.

The couple's nightmare began the night they decided to leave, and their destiny changed forever, leaving them with deep scars, which seem to still be bleeding.

Refugees Who Become a Couple and Family in Exile

Some refugee families are families which have been composed in England, where each couple member brings with them their past experiences of having had to leave their home country behind. Nadia and Akbar are not married; they lived together for 16 years and have broken up now but remain very close friends. They both wanted to be part of my interviews, as they each felt that their past experiences had contributed to them splitting up after so long. The couple met in England after having fled Afghanistan; they do not have children. Both Akbar and Nadia were politically active against the Taliban regime, so the phase of pre-flight was a very difficult one for them each individually. They were not yet a couple during this phase and so do not have any shared lived experiences, although they each express the same sense of being victim to violence and oppression.

Akbar was politically active in Afghanistan as part of a communist party from his 20s, and they fought against the Taliban regime. He therefore had a very unusual life of living in the woods and mountains, constantly in hiding. He described how, at first, they were strong and could fight against the Taliban; however, after a few years they were being killed and destroyed, until in the end Akbar had to run away, as his life was in serious danger.

> *The Taliban regime used to execute all oppositional people. This is why we had to be at war against them because otherwise we would get killed. Many of my friends were killed. 'Islam' killed one of my best friends as he was standing right next to me. Other friends were executed and hung. All my youth I had fought against Muslims. I had spent a lifetime at war with Islam.*

Akbar spoke of the difficult times he and his family endured after the Taliban came to power.

> *The Taliban used to come into our home unannounced to search the house to see if we were hiding people there; sometimes they would come several times a day, up to seven times. Yes, at all times of the day and night, first at midnight, then at 3 a.m. and then again at 5 a.m. So, we lived a very different life to before the Taliban came to power. The resistance went on for many years, and I was shot twice. We would fight in the hills and mountains, and sometimes through the night, and one time I got lost and didn't really know*

where I was, we were three people. I had been shot, and it took us 18 days to find our way back to the base camp again.

Akbar also described how the Taliban coming into power had made a change in his family and other families around him.

You know, during that time, there was a revolution in each and every family around Afghanistan as well. Just imagine this kind of radical thinking together with politics getting mixed in our home, it was like dynamite! All my siblings were fighters and part of the resistance; we all carried weapons in our war against the Taliban regime, even my sisters. The whole family had become political and activist. If certain family members had different political opinion to ours, we would not keep in touch.

I remember the first anti-Taliban leaflet I saw; I took it home and had hidden it under a chest in my room. My mum had seen it and asked me why I had hidden it under the chest. I explained to her that it was forbidden; she wondered why, and I said that it was political, and she asked me to read it to her, as she was illiterate. Afterwards she asked me to always bring any other political leaflets home and to read them to her and give them to her so that she could keep them for me. After that I would always share all the political information I had with her, and we would start to discuss politics, world news and so on together. I remember we always had the photo of an activist in our home; my mother was extremely opposed to injustice and dictatorship, and this had a great influence on all of my siblings and me.

Nadia was living in England when the Taliban were coming into power, and she went back to Afghanistan against her family's wishes. She soon became politically active and was finally arrested and sent to prison.

So many of the young generation were fighting against the Taliban regime and for freedom of speech, freedom of opinions and freedom of not wearing the hijab. I remember we demonstrated against the hijab, and they attacked us, hit us and all the rest. Three years later I was arrested. I was in prison for eight years, and I was supposed to be executed, but my father had certain contacts and he changed the verdict so that they wouldn't kill me; all of my friends were executed, though. All my friends were executed. After I came out of prison, I stayed in Afghanistan for three years, and during these three years I was constantly under surveillance, and it was getting ridiculous. They wanted to put pressure on me. There is so much pressure on you, so much persecution that you feel like screaming!! In the end, I decided to leave; it was too risky. I was limited and controlled and in danger of being arrested again.

Nadia did not really speak about her past before going to prison, as if she could not remember the Nadia before prison. I recall asking her to tell me about her life before and, after a moment's hesitation, she spoke of herself as a very stubborn and strong-headed child:

> *In my family, I was born after three boys, my brothers; I had to be strong enough to stand up to them for my rights, and I became strong and resilient from that. I also think I am definitely the granddaughter of my paternal grandmother because she was a very strong woman. At present, I can't even pretend to be the person I used to be, and I have learnt to accept that I am very different now. Many people find it hard to accept themselves as changed and want to go back to the way they were before prison, but I worked on myself to accept myself the way I am now. I allow myself to isolate myself; I don't fight with myself.*

Akbar spoke with regret about his past identity.

> *Before, I used to be so decisive, so independent, in every possible way—in society, in the resistance, amongst friends, financially. I never had to ask for help; on the contrary, people would come to me for help. People always used to say about me that I used to laugh a lot and that that is why I have such a wide mouth. Before I came to the West you could not see me without laughter on my lips, despite the conflicts.*

Both Akbar and Nadia have spent their lives in resistance and have shown a great deal of resilience. Nadia spoke about her time in prison:

> *I started to work on myself even when I was in prison because I soon realised what prison was doing to me and others around me. I decided that when I got out, I would learn music because I knew that music is healing and learning music would feed my soul but also help me get my concentration skills and learning skills back. Even in prison I read as much as I possibly could, no matter what the book was. I kept my mind busy at all times in prison, and when I came out, I started to study music (in secret) the three years I was in Afghanistan, and it really helped me, it saved me.*
> *Just imagine that when we were in prison, they would take our friend to be executed, you knew it and you heard the shot, so you know your friend has been executed but you do NOT cry, you show no emotion whatsoever because the guards are watching you and want to see you suffer and you know this and don't want to give them satisfaction. You therefore learn to never show emotion of any kind.*

Akbar had status in his role in the resistance, and this is something he is proud of.

They were each forced to leave Afghanistan and seek refuge in Europe in order not to be killed.

Flight

Despite having worked for so many years with refugees, I am still shaken when I hear what refugees go through to get to a 'safe' host country. Their stories are so varied, but all are full of feelings of fear, hopelessness and helplessness; they are also an ode to the refugees' courage in not giving up and continuing to fight, showing determination to have a safer life.

Although Fatemeh and her son, Rooh, came to England with a visa, leaving Iraq to join her husband meant being brutally forced to leave her life behind, her family and friends, where she was unable to tell her mother or to say goodbye.

> *We were so frightened at the airport, so scared of being found out. Every time they checked our passports at the airport in Iraq we were petrified. No one knew, no one said goodbye; I cannot forget that I never said goodbye to my mother, that I did not get to kiss her face.*

I cannot help but remember when I was a 13-year-old girl at the airport, feeling sick with pain for leaving Iran and wondering whether I would ever see my friends again. Hearing Fatemeh tell her story of forced separation, I become that young girl who was never given the opportunity to say goodbye to my friends and family, to prepare myself for the great loss I was going to suffer.

Mahdi remembered his journey to England with little emotion and explained that compared to the hardships he had suffered in Iraq, the journey to freedom was not even comparable.

> *I went from town to town, hiding, and left Iraq to Turkey and from there to England. The journey by land was very hard, from Iraq to Turkey especially. We were without food or water for four days, and in general we were often without food and water. I could feel that outside of Iraq, people, even family, had to think of themselves first, and the kind of solidarity we had before was no longer there. I felt I couldn't count on my own brother in Germany because he was in no position to help me; I had to only count on myself.*

For Tina, Hamed and their two sons, the journey to England was a nightmare which haunts them still. Like most of my clients, they came with the help of smugglers; however, these smugglers and fellow countrymen were abusive towards the vulnerable families they were supposed to be helping.

> *The smugglers would frighten us and tell us that if we left the house we would be arrested and sent back to Afghanistan; we were scared, and we stayed indoors all the time. One time the smuggler took us to a house where there was no electricity, water, or heating in the cold winter, with just one mattress on the floor. One other time we were with a smuggler who used to smoke marijuana and we had to share a small studio with him. The studio would fill*

up with his marijuana smoke, and I was afraid for my boys. His mood also changed regularly, and he was very nasty to us, shouting, being rude; it was horrible. The smuggler said he had to send us to England separately. We had to listen to him, or he would just abandon us. They lose interest in you when you get arrested a couple of times, you are no longer profitable.

Tina and her family went back and forth between France, Belgium, Germany and Holland, trying to get to England with their fake passports. Tina recounted how they were arrested on several occasions at various airports and taken to camps because their fake passports were of poor quality.

There was nothing I could do but to do as the smuggler said, even if he made me go to the different airports 50 times with fear, stress and so forth; I had to do it, I had no choice. The police took me and the boys to a refugee camp; my husband was taken somewhere else. You know I think the officials at the airports could see the fright on my and my son's faces and that made them suspect us more. One time they took me and my husband to prison and the children to like an orphanage. You cannot imagine the panic and fright of these two young children. We weren't even told for how long or anything.

Whilst they were in hiding in the different countries in Europe, they had to be careful not to be seen by the police. However, the police almost always found out about them and took them away to refugee camps.

We were so frightened. If we went out, maybe twice, my husband would go out first and then we would sneak out so that the neighbours wouldn't see us and call the police. My youngest son would panic when he saw policemen and shout 'Let's run! Let's run!'

Hamed spoke with great emotion about their traumatic journey to the United Kingdom and needed to speak in detail about it.

We suffered so many difficulties on our journey from Afghanistan. We fled from Afghanistan to Tajikistan. We came to France, and after that it was hell. We went to Belgium because the smuggler we knew was based in Belgium, and we stayed there for 50 days. Out of these 50 days, 30 days we spent in a studio flat which was a few metres big, where we slept huddled up with my wife and two sons in the living room. We had no blankets, it was dirty, there was no heating, and this was the month of January, it was freezing. The smuggler took us to a house and said no one should know we were living there so we couldn't come and go as we wanted; we were in hiding all the time. From there he took us to Holland. It was a nightmare in Holland; the smuggler took us to different houses. We stayed for about two weeks with him, and he kept saying every day that he would help us leave but then nothing happened.

As Hamed remembered the number of times they were caught out and taken away by the police, his body tensed, his back hunched, until he almost held his head in his hands.

The police took our sons to a foster home and put my wife and I in jail; they treated us extremely badly, so verbally abusive and rude; there were no human rights. They took us to jail, and we had no idea what was going to happen to us; we were petrified and imagined all sorts of things. Imagine the children's fear! We were so frightened, but imagine the fright of our children! The smuggler later took us to France, and we tried to take the plane to England from there but were obviously caught. I kept asking them to take me to a doctor for the excruciating pain in my back, but they wouldn't listen.

Hamed went on to tell me that not only did they keep getting arrested but the smugglers became more abusive with every arrest, and as time went on, the family were more and more at their mercy.

After we were set free the smuggler took us to another house which belonged to a friend of his. We had to wait outside in the freezing cold for five hours until 10 p.m. for him to bring the key. When we went into the house it was completely empty, there wasn't even a lamp. The owner then came and wanted to kick us out; she could see we had two young boys, but she had no mercy. My younger son was in his underwear but kept saying, 'let's run before they get us, let's run.' He looked petrified. The smuggler then took us to a house where there was no water, and I had to carry water for us from outside. The smuggler also had other passengers staying in another flat; he used to take the food I bought for my family and would sell it to his other passengers. Because we needed him, I couldn't protest or say anything. The smuggler was no longer interested in helping us get to England because it was difficult, so we went into so much trouble to get in touch with him; he had taken our money! We went to Belgium with a new smuggler, who told us we couldn't all go to England together, we had to go separately, me first and then my wife and children together.

They had to listen to the smuggler and Hamed came to England first while Tina and the boys struggled for another two months, going from one airport to the next to try and come to England with their fake passports.

Hamed was arrested at the airport in England and taken to prison.

When I arrived in England the officer had suspicions about my passport. They arrested me at the airport here, and I was in prison for six months. This prison was terrible where we only had permission to go out into the fresh air once per week for 20 minutes. My six-month sentence had to finish on the 19th of October, and I was counting the days, but they kept stalling although legally my six-month sentence had finished. I had been counting the days to be free. They kept saying my bail wasn't ready and that it was my lawyer's fault. This dragged on for another ten days. I had had enough because I was now only in prison for administrative reasons.

Throughout their ordeal, however, the couple were able to be resilient, and Tina remembered how she and her husband had stood up to the smugglers at times and, for example, gone out to buy essentials for their children or how she had argued with one smuggler who had gotten them arrested numerous times because of the poor quality of their fake passports. Tina also resisted the police in various countries and ran away from the camps she was placed in a few times. She had to keep on reassuring and comforting her sons during their ordeal together and despite all the difficulties, she managed to stay positive and hopeful for her sons; she did not lose her calm and was able to think clearly under all the stress in order to keep her family safe. '*I knew from my husband's experience that we should not enter the UK with passports, so we tore them up, with so much stress, so much stress in the plane.*' Tina looked at me with a smile and said: '*You know, I've lost everything, but I still have a lot of intelligence.*'

Hamed was less able to talk about times when he had shown resilience, and I had a real sense of his feelings of helplessness when he spoke of their flight. I think this may be because he felt a failure as a protective figure in his family, that he could not protect his family the way he wanted to. However, he was always also able to keep his sons in mind. '*The children were very distressed, and my wife and I kept joking with them to make them more relaxed.*' Hamed did, nevertheless, speak with pride about one time when he had fought off two thieves at a train station in Belgium:

As we were getting on the train, I felt a man pulling at my bag, the bag had all our money in it, and I wasn't going to let them have it. I was badly hurt with a broken finger, but I had managed to save all our money from getting stolen. I also hurt my back and suffered from back pain for months after that, but they didn't get our money.

I think for me, the difficulties that Pooneh and Siavash endured seem even more unbearable, as they did not even really need to leave Iran; they were young and made a hasty decision to leave, mostly out of pride for Siavash, (a sense of wanting to live independently from his intrusive family) and Pooneh followed because of her love for him. She had lived such a loving and protected life until then, and the devastating events which followed their decision to leave have had an immense negative impact on them and their lives today.

Pooneh was animated when she remembered how vulnerable she had felt leaving Iran and having to put all her trust in a stranger (smuggler), being at this person's mercy.

The woman smuggler kept delaying, and she had taken our passports already with a large amount of money, and every document we had was in her hands.

In the end she came and said there was a change of plans and she could not take us directly to France but that we had to go to Kyrgyzstan first and then on from there. We felt stuck and extremely vulnerable because she had our passports and she had taken our money, so we felt we had no choice but to do as she said. When we got to Kyrgyzstan, she said, 'actually you're not going straight to France; you will have to stay here for two weeks.' My God, we just couldn't imagine what was going to happen to us, and she had all our belongings!

When Pooneh and her husband arrived in Kyrgyzstan, they realised they had to live with a dozen young men refugees. Pooneh felt very insecure, as she was the only young woman amongst all these men. The men were being smuggled out because they were criminals and were trying to avoid jail; they were dangerous and stole Pooneh and Siavash's laptops and cameras and various other things the first few days they were there.

During these two weeks, if I ever went to the bathroom, my husband would come with me and stand outside, that's how much danger there was for me with all these violent men sharing the house with us. On the second day they had a huge fight, and one hit the other with a knife and there was blood everywhere.

Pooneh's ordeal had just started, as they were now told that they could no longer go directly to France from Kyrgyzstan. They had to first fly to Russia and from there to Germany. Then, they were told, they would be on their own.

They said when you land in Germany, you are on your own, and that's it. We were left with nothing, what were we going to do in Germany? If they were to arrest us, that would be the end for us, we had to get through. We were so frightened.

When they went through the customs and were 'free', the reality of their situation became even more real; they were on their own.

We came out from the airport in Dusseldorf and felt lost, what were we to do, where to go? We had entered with fake passports, and my husband was afraid of being caught out and we were just both insecure and scared.

They decided it would be safer to take the train to Paris and avoid airports. Siavash's aunt lived in Paris, and she advised them to not stay in France but to go to England because the government in France was being extremely strict on illegal immigrants.

My husband's aunt said she would find us someone to take us to Calais and then smuggle us over to England. The man came and told us we would be leaving the next day. When we arrived in Calais, we asked him, so where do we stay? He said, 'nowhere but on this beach, out in the open'. He said we had to stay there until he found us a way to go over, and he didn't know how long it would take. We saw that people were already basically living there, in cardboard boxes, on the beach. They were all waiting to someday go over to England. It was so very terrifying. We couldn't sleep; we didn't dare to close our eyes for even a second. At night, the smuggler said to us that he was going to try and find a way to smuggle us over. He showed us a huge truck and told me to crawl under on my stomach, get inside through a tiny hole. I was sobbing and said I couldn't do it. He said there were already 20 other people in the place who had gone through the hole. I just sobbed and refused to crawl under the truck and go into the unknown like that. He said I had to do it and that it would take us three days to get to England. Three days in a truck with 20 people I didn't know, under such terrible conditions. I refused.

Then the French police came to arrest them along with the other refugees waiting to come over to England.

They took us and a few others and took us to the police station. At first, they put us all in a tiny cell with 30 other people and we were so cramped up! The police treated us so very badly; they humiliated us, swore at us and one time I was holding a cloth to my nose because of the unbearable smell in the cell and a policeman said to me: 'what are you trying not to smell? This is your own stink!'

Because Siavash spoke fluent French, they were soon released. The couple realised they could not rely on the smuggler to help them across the border and decided to go to Holland and try to come to England via Holland. They arrived in Norwich and from there went to Glasgow, where they had family. However, the couple still had even harder times to follow. Pooneh recounts:

We lived in Glasgow for eight months, but they refused to give us refugee status, and because we were childless they were going to take everything away from us; they took away the flat, we had no permit to work and we were given a week to be deported. So, after eight months in Glasgow, the police kicked us out, my God, what were we going to do now? My husband said we should try to go to Canada, just emigrate there. As if all the horror we had gone through wasn't enough! So again, we had to get out our old fake passports; we went to Dublin to try and go from there. But when we tried to get on a plane to Canada, they arrested us. They took us to a refugee camp in Dublin. The police confiscated everything and took us to the refugee camp with nothing. I then found out I was eight weeks pregnant! It was as if my whole world, what was left of it, crumbled around me. The last thing I wanted was for my child to be born in such conditions, in a camp!

Pooneh and Siavash stayed at the camp for three and a half months, after which they were sent back to England and were sent to Leeds; they stayed in Leeds for four years, where their daughter was born. The family were left in limbo for many years, without a response about their refugee status. As Pooneh describes:

> *They kept us without a response for four years! No work permits, no hope of a future, in temporary refugee housing, but thank goodness at least in England you get a flat; you don't have to live in a camp. I had left Iran with such a high education, had had such a good and rich professional life, so much experience and such a desire to work, and yet I couldn't, as if I was stuck in a swamp for five years, pulling me down. As soon as we got a driver's licence, they interrogated us about that. What terrible interrogations, so degrading. Our family sent us money to buy a car, and it became a problem and again we had to explain where we had gotten the money for the car; in the end we sold it. I had earned good money in Iran, and now I had to answer to them.*

Although Pooneh remembered these difficult times with sadness, it was clear to me that she had put it in the past and was much more focused on her present life and career and on building a future for herself and her family. It is as if the hardship Pooneh went through was a motivation for her to make sure she is never in a position again of feeling humiliated by authorities because of her dependency on them.

Siavash, on the other hand, seemed to be stuck in the past. He was extremely emotional during the interview and remembered their sense of vulnerability with his whole being.

> *Those first 15 days of journey to Europe were the most horrific days of my life; I will never forget them. We were told 48 hours before that we had to leave Iran, so we only had 48 hours to pack our things and be ready. I didn't sleep for these 48 hours. The first night we arrived in Kyrgyzstan, they took us to a four- bedroom house where we were supposed to stay, all 15 of us; my wife and I and 13 young men. The other 13 were not from the same background as us; they had never left Iran, and they used to get drunk every night and get into fights.*

Siavash recounted their stay in Calais with deep pain.

> *We slept in boxes like the homeless, but mostly we stayed awake and walked the whole time, day and night; the smugglers wanted to get us over during the night, so we had to walk and wait for them to signal us at any moment. Then as soon as it was daytime the police would come to check the place, so we couldn't sleep then either. The only time I remember sleeping without fear for a few moments while in Calais was when we were so exhausted that we decided to sleep in a public toilet, one of those automatic ones you pay to go*

*into. We slept there for about an hour, but then the alarm of the toilet went off
because it has a limit to how long you can stay in there. The smugglers themselves were vicious and dangerous people. I was so afraid that they would
do something to my wife. I was so stressed the whole time. Many times, the
families would be split up and sent separately, it was so difficult. I was very
afraid that they would try to split me and my wife up and send us separately.
You are also in a situation where you cannot say no to the smugglers. You are
not in a position to make any decisions; you just have to obey.*

Siavash blamed himself for having made the decision to come to England,
especially as they were denied refugee status the first time.

*We therefore made an even more stupid and childish decision than the first
one to come to England; we decided to go to Canada. Our decision to go
to Canada was the start of an even bigger nightmare than our journey to
England. We went to Ireland with our fake passports to fly to Canada from
there. We didn't want to fly from England because if we got caught, they
would have put us in prison. All our documents for Canada were ready; we
had again paid a lot of money to a person to get them forged and ready. As
soon as the official saw our passports, he said he was suspicious and called
his supervisor to come. We had to wait for two hours, but they couldn't
find anything wrong with the passports, and we went through to the Irish
immigration check to be questioned. They separated us and interviewed us
separately for three hours. The police wanted to put us in prison until we
agreed to give our true identity, and during these three to four hours we
went through so much anxiety; my wife just cried and cried the whole time
and trembled. We declared ourselves as refugees, and they put us in a camp
instead of prison.*

Although England had denied the couple refugee status because it was the first
country in which they had applied for asylum, the British authorities had to accept
them back. Now that they were expecting a child and their circumstances had
changed, and they were coming back to England from a different country, they
could ask for asylum again. They therefore declared themselves as refugees at the
airport in England.

*We waited for almost five years to get an answer from the authorities. Wait-
ing means that you cannot work, ever; you are just allowed to live like a
vegetable and get benefits and basically not have a life; you slowly die. They
put so much pressure on you that a lot of people just decide to go back to
their home country themselves. They had given us a flat and we also received
£60 per week. You cannot imagine how difficult the wait was; to have to wait
a year and a half after my wife's first interview to even hear anything, every
day of this one and a half years I waited for the post, anxiously, nervously, it*

was a daily torture. We waited for five years altogether. Five years of mental and emotional torture.

I think it is always important to draw out the strength and resilience of refugees in all stages of their flight, and I am in awe of Pooneh's psychological strength throughout their ordeal because she never gave up becoming the person she wanted to be again; she never forgot where she had come from and who she was.

Day and night my thoughts were about how I could escape from my situation, our situation, how can I get back into society, be a part of something, be a person again? I was determined to get back my old life, my old self; and then to improve. I kept on planning for the future and knew exactly what I would do the day after I received my leave to remain. That's why I studied, worked voluntarily; I had planned everything. It had to happen, it just had to.

According to Pooneh, the reason the family were given leave to remain was because she had kept them in the loop of all her voluntary work in a lawyer's office working with immigrants, how she had studied up to level two of the immigration advisory and she had also passed her IELTS exam with excellent results. Pooneh said with pride that the Home Office sent them a letter to say that they had chosen certain citizens who were well integrated to give leave to remain to.

Siavash showed resilience during their difficult journey to England, keeping his wife safe at any cost, but he seemed to give up once they came to England the second time. He recounted how he just waited and waited for an answer from the Home Office, getting more and more desperate and deflated. He did not keep active in any way and did not even learn English during the wait. His description of his state of mind at the time makes me think he was depressed and unable to pull himself together. Maybe the guilt of having put his wife in such a dire situation stopped him from doing anything productive.

Nadia's journey to the United Kingdom was rather uneventful, and she recounted feeling safe very quickly. She booked a flight from Afghanistan to Germany via London, and she had decided to get off in London and seek asylum at the airport. Her sister lived here and had already engaged a lawyer for her. As Nadia got off the plane, she described how frightened she was walking towards the passport control area. She was so nervous that when she saw an official at the airport, she went up to him and said: '*I am seeking asylum, help me.*' Unfortunately, the official did not respond in the way she expected.

He said 'we don't want refugees', and he pushed my passport back into my hand!! He would not let me go any further, and he kept me in the corridor and was physically pushing me backwards towards the planes and away from the passport controls. He kept saying go back to your country, and I knew if he forced me to go back, I would be executed for sure this time. I don't know how

I managed, but it was a matter of life and death and I managed to get away from him and started to run towards the passport controls as he ran after me.

For Akbar, the phase of flight was more difficult, although as he himself told me, the difficulties were not comparable to what he had been through in Afghanistan. Akbar had to leave the party's base in Iraq because his life was in danger there as well. He fled to Turkey, but he soon realised he was being watched even there.

I was in hiding in Turkey, but the Taliban regime had killed so many of my friends that I feared they would be able to find me even there. I could never go out during the day; I lived in constant fear of getting killed.

During their interviews, each person spoke about the changes they see in themselves and in their partner and how the family dynamics had changed because of the adverse experiences they had been through as described earlier. I therefore asked them to speak to me about these changes in more depth and shall be sharing them under the title 'Post-Flight', looking at the effects of the lived trauma on each of the partners individually and then in their couple relationship.

Post-Flight Effects of Trauma on Individual Family Members

Fatemeh and Mahdi are expecting a baby and therefore have plans for their future, but they are also highly aware of the changes in themselves and each other due to all the trauma and difficulties.

Fatemeh described the way their life in Iraq had affected Rooh, their son; witnessing the Secret Service coming, on numerous occasions, to take his father or mother away for interrogations, and later seeing his father disappear without any explanation.

To this day Rooh asks his father if he is going to stay with us and not disappear again. Even now whenever someone knocks on the door, he gets very frightened, so does my husband. We suddenly think we are in Iraq . . . the Secret Service are knocking on our door. They are going to capture my husband and take him away. When someone knocks on the door, we automatically say: 'They're here' like we always said in Iraq, 'They're here!' My husband's state is even worse than me; still to this day he never stays in the flat on his own. He is too afraid, and so is our son.'

Fatemeh spoke of her own sufferings:

I cry so often. I cannot feel any joy, no smile on my face; I am just sad. When I lived in Iraq, I lived in constant fear, but here I live in constant sadness and feel the loss of my family. I cannot really feel joy anymore. I cannot forget the difficulties of the past and move on. I have not had any problems in England, but I have been very depressed. I know I should be happy to be out of Iraq and safe, finally, but I cannot understand why I cannot feel any joy.

In my clinical experience, this seems to be a common theme; my clients feel guilty about feeling depressed now that they are safe and should be feeling relief and a sense of freedom. The refugees I work with almost all describe how they are confused about why they feel so low in the UK. I believe it is because until they get leave to remain and feel safe, they are in survival mode and are fighting to keep alive and reach their goal of getting permission to stay in the host country, fighting all the adversity they face. Once they are safe, the past trauma almost hits them and they feel confused, depressed and they show signs of PTSD.

It is as if Fatemeh almost blames herself for not being able to forget about her past traumas and be happy in England, where she is safe. And yet, it is beyond her control: '*It's as if I cannot get empty enough. It is all in me, still here [pointing to her heart]. It is in us now. We are like a broken vase that cannot be put back together again.*' Fatemeh's use of 'we' and 'us' where she includes her husband and son in her declarations shows that she is aware of the way the past has affected all three of them.

Mahdi spoke in detail about the physical and emotional damage the traumas of his past have had on him.

In prison, they paid me a lesson which leaves me deaf to this day. I remember when I had come out of prison, I was constantly afraid, and whenever they knocked on the door I would run away. I would get panic attacks when I heard a noise; even now this continues. I had never gotten on a plane before they took me to Baghdad that time, and to this day I associate airplanes with torture. I cannot hear or see a plane without having flashbacks from my terrible experiences. I go back to that time and the fear and anxiety comes back, just from hearing a plane! I try to tell myself it's the past, but it really isn't. Another example is that as soon as I see a policeman here, I feel extremely fearful; even if I know the police have a protective role here. It's not what I know logically; it's beyond my control this fear I feel, this fear of being caught and taken away by them. I often have flashbacks during the day and always, always nightmares. It all paralyses me. I keep having constant fears, and I cannot control them; if I hear the door, if people are walking behind me, if I am alone, these are very difficult things to deal with on a daily basis. In Iraq, every time I went out, I was afraid I would get arrested, tortured, killed, but I never felt depressed, the depression I feel here is new to me. I don't understand why.

Mahdi then told me something which made me realise that his torture is ongoing through the doubt the torturers have put into his mind:

One of my tortures was that they used to inject me with different things, and now I get terrible dizziness all the time and fall; I don't know what they injected in me, maybe it's that. I also get extremely angry for no reason which

I didn't before. I try to control myself, but I can feel the anger, and sometimes I can throw things out of anger.

Many other refugees I work with live in constant fear of being exposed by their torturers, as in countries such as Afghanistan, Iraq and Syria; incidents of torture are filmed, with the threat of being put online. Many of the incidents of torture include sexual acts, and when refugees (men and women) find that they can trust me, they tell me that they are constantly checking online to see if they are being exposed. They are thus continuously tortured, feeling that it will never end.

Mahdi is aware of the influence of generational stories on himself and his own family:

From the day I was born I have lived in fear because my father and older brothers were all politically active. Once when I went to see my GP, he asked me if I knew what happiness is, and I said I don't think I have ever really felt it. I may have laughed sometimes, but I have never really felt happy, really felt it.

Tina spoke about the effects of the traumas the family had suffered on her sons.

I can see the effect of the past traumas on my older son in his character a lot. He is extremely, extremely short tempered now and very nervous, you wouldn't believe it. You know, coming here, immigration, the difficulties we've been through getting here, the difficulties we have here, losing everything, losing our loved ones; all of these were a very difficult part of the boys' lives. My younger son is so unhappy; he is just tearful all the time. My younger son never used to bed wet as a child, now he bed wets even now. He never speaks, in general is extremely quiet. He is 11 and was 8 when we came. Sometimes I go to his room and see him crying, and no matter what I do to get him to talk to me he remains quiet. I took them to see a family therapist, and I went with them; my husband refused to come with us and said he needed help for himself first. They did not say a word to the therapist, even if I encouraged them and opened up about our past and present difficulties; they did not say a word. In the end the therapist said she could not force them to see her.

Tina also shared her worry for her husband and the changes she sees in him. '*I feel that after his sister's death, he has become very depressed. I mean he is very . . . no I mean he WAS sociable, really, past tense.*'

With this linguistic mistake, Tina suddenly became very sad, as if she remembered the past vividly and could see her sociable and confident husband in her mind. I waited silently, and after a while she smiled and wiped her tears and continued:

He has become cold and indifferent after his sister's death, as if he takes no pleasure in anything. I feel he is not concerned about anything anymore. My husband always says that he may forget a lot of things but that he can never forget our sons' fright that night, when the police again raided the house we were hiding in.

Tina spoke with great regret and emotion about how the past traumas have affected her:

I will never forget that the rape happened on the last days of my period, and every time I have my period I get re-traumatised. Last time I went to my GP and said, 'give me something so that I never have to have my period again.' I can never get rid of the Taliban's stink in my nose, it is always there. He had had lunch before and had eaten onions, and even to this day I cannot stand the sight or smell of onions; I go crazy. I can't stand the smell of airports either. I just prefer to isolate myself, be in my own world. Even if my son kisses me and he is unshaved, I get very anxious because the sheikh had not shaved either. Once my boys had a physical fight and I saw my older son standing almost on his brother on the sofa. I cried so much; I just couldn't stand it. I cannot take it when someone is being forced to do something because he is not strong. It just reminded me of the man and how he had forced me to accept things and do things because I had no choice. I am so depressed, so changed, always taking medications. I am so broken that there is nothing left of me. Sometimes when I walk in the house I want to just fight, I want to moan and groan about things to start an argument, and when I start I don't want to stop. Someone said to me to go to Europe on holiday with the family, but I said to her that when I hear the word 'Europe' I tremble all over.

Hamed only spoke briefly about the effects of the traumatic experiences on his sons. I don't know if this is because it was too painful for him or if it is because he has too many difficulties himself to hold his sons' pain in mind.

For a long time, every time my son saw a policeman he became terribly stressed and had panic attacks. Unfortunately, the children are both dam- aged from the past, everything I have told you. So unfortunate. They are both aggressive, short fused and nervous. My oldest is impossible, so extremely tense all the time. They are constantly fighting with each other.

Hamed did not say much about his traumatic experiences during their flight to England and spoke mostly about his experiences in prison in England.

I was in the prison and after two weeks I reacted and self-harmed and didn't eat for days. It was when I heard about my sister's death. But I really lost it when my prison sentence was over, and I still had to stay there for an extra ten days because my paperwork was delayed. I lost it; I felt like I was going mad. They took me to an isolation cell, and I broke every piece of furniture there was in the cell; I had completely lost my mind, it was all too much. I tried to cut my veins to bleed to death; I just wanted to die.

This statement clearly shows how bureaucracy and paperwork can have such a seriously detrimental effect on a human being's life. Hamed had every right to leave prison, yet he was forced to stay in jail an extra ten days while his paperwork was being prepared, and these extra ten days just drove him to a state of complete despair after all the difficulties he had already endured.

I am not the same person; I used to be extremely confident, independent and limitless. For me, after all the difficulties and after having lost my sister because of my mistakes, life has no meaning anymore, there is no going back.

Pooneh got a very good job a week after she was given leave to remain and is successful in her work. Although this job has nothing to do with her qualifications as a nutritionist, she has excelled in her new role. Pooneh said her new life and happiness have helped her to not think of the past, although she did say she still has nightmares about some of her past experiences. Pooneh was, however, concerned for her husband. '*He still hasn't adapted at all. He is still very low, hopeless, and depressed. I feel with time he is getting worse, more depressed and more critical.*'

I remember feeling concerned for Siavash during and even after the interview because there was a deep sense of sadness and hopelessness in him.

I always said to myself that the day I would get leave to remain would be the happiest day of my life, but I was too drained to feel much, I had been through too much. Of course, I was happy, but I couldn't feel the exhilaration I imagined I would feel. I just felt numb. Even though our trip from Iran was difficult, we had a goal, a purpose, but when you fail in your goal, you just lose all hope, you feel such a failure. These five years mean to me that I have no hope of ever feeling happy again; it has brought me down to my knees. The pain never goes away, the wounds never heal. I think I cannot remember what being happy feels like.

Despite all the difficult experiences the couple lived through, it is clear that Siavash was most affected by the five years they had to wait for a response from the Home Office.

Akbar spoke with emotion about the changes in him. '*When I came out from Afghanistan, I stopped smiling and laughing, as if I had dried up. I did not laugh again, to this day.*'

He recounted how he still felt fearful after having lived in safety in Sweden for several months:

I was still traumatised and felt insecure. I'll never forget when I started learning Swedish and the teacher called out my name on the first day of the course,

I did not answer her to let her know it was me. By this time, I had already been in Sweden for seven months! I went after the class and asked the teacher to call me by a different name because I didn't feel safe.

Then Akbar shared with me his hatred and fear of Islam, and I began to understand more why he had said, earlier in the interview, that he had fought Islam all his life and not the Taliban regime.

I remember when I came to London, many years later, I embarked in the east of London, and I was in a hostel, there used to be an Islamic centre nearby, and instead of walking past the Islamic centre to go home, I used to go around the whole block to avoid the Islamic centre because I was so very afraid. I said to myself that Muslims were there and all my youth I had fought against Muslims, and ever since then, whenever I hear someone is calling themselves Muslim, I get a bad, anxious feeling. Would you believe me if I told you that it has still, to this day, not faded, this fear I have of Islam and Muslims? I still feel anxious, as anxious as before. I feel very insecure around people who call themselves Muslims. I know logically that a mosque is a very natural place where people go not only to pray but also to gather, talk, etc., but my emotions take over my logic and I feel scared and insecure and anxious. For example, where I work, we have a voluntary worker, who is called Islam, he is from Chechnya. He looks nice, but when I heard his name, I immediately felt a sense of hatred towards him. I said to him to be patient with me and explained that I had spent a lifetime at war with Islam, that I still have a bullet from Islam in my leg and that I am still physically and mentally damaged by Islam. I also feel that I get irritated much faster than I should, that I feel aggressive, I get angry very fast. I have very little tolerance.

Akbar concluded by saying:

You know, when you have been through hardships, it's as if you get layers of distress laying like dust on you and you need help to shake it off every now and again. These layers affect your character, your life, and they show themselves from time to time; I notice them now and again.

Although Nadia had been quite mask faced and smiley during the interview, she showed more emotion when she spoke about how the past traumas have affected her. She no longer laughed and was quite pensive and almost quiet in her voice.

I think no one really understands what prison and the experiences we have had in prison do to us. It has impacted my life forever, and of course it has a huge impact on any relationship I may have with a man. I don't think anyone can really understand what prison has done to me and others like me. I know that even if I have done a lot of work on myself, there are a lot of the damages that will stay with me until I am dead, and I shall take them to the grave with me. It changed my character completely; I was very sociable, had a lot of friends, close friends, but after prison I isolate myself, I don't socialise. When I was in prison, I could feel myself changing, and I knew that I was being damaged; I couldn't think, I couldn't concentrate, etc. Also, in never showing any emotion, it's as if I wore a mask for eight years, and even now I cannot really take off the mask; it is part of me. Psychologically it has had a huge impact on me, but physically as well; I am registered as being disabled even if it is not obvious. I was so distressed and shocked, but the GP explained that my body was too damaged to do physical work of any kind.

I am too weak and damaged physically to have children. That is why I write books because each book is like a child to me, as I can never have any children. The torture and pressure were so intensive in prison that I cannot remember a lot of my life before prison. It's as if the 8 years in prison have crushed back the 23 years of my life before it. I often think about all the things in my life that I have forgotten about, that they have washed out of my mind and soul.

Nadia concluded that she no longer suffers from flashbacks and nightmares like she used to and believes that her writing has helped her.

Effects of Trauma on Family Relationships

With regard to her relationship to her son, Fatemeh says, with regret in her voice:

I am quite intolerant, get angry quickly. I am very depressed. I have no patience anymore. I want to stay in my room, isolate myself. I just put a blanket over my head and think about my family, about the past. I don't want to get angry with my son, but I often feel I don't really feel like talking to him, spending time with him. When he sees me crying, he tries to comfort me.

This last statement shows how family structures can change in times of hardship and how Rooh may be taking on the role of carer for his parents, who are both suffering from depression and anxiety. It also makes me wonder how isolated Rooh might be, with two parents who, as much as they try, cannot seem to find enough space in their minds to be present with their son.

Mahdi was also very aware of the effects the past difficulties and traumatic events have had and still have on him as a father and a husband.

This affects my family life in a bad way. It has not been good. We were both under so much mental pressure all the time, my wife and I in Iraq. She saw them take me away, she has seen everything, but she still doesn't know what they did to me in prison. I have told her a bit but not everything. Sometimes she asks about my time in prison, and I have told her very little because I couldn't keep completely quiet about it.

It saddens me to see the silence the hardships have caused between this couple who care for each other so much; there are things which are just too painful to share and talk about. Mahdi describes the distance this creates within his relationships.

> *I was never very present for my wife; I was either caught up in my activities or caught up in my fears. I therefore never really felt close to my wife or child; there is a distance between us because they don't know all that I've been through, and I don't want them to know. I am unhappy about this; I am unhappy with myself. My political activities have had such a negative impact on my family, immediate and larger family. Our whole family has been pulled apart.*

Mahdi is also worried about the effects the past has had on his son and on their father–son relationship:

> *Even my son has been affected and me as a father; I love people and I try to be kind to them, but I don't have much patience or much joy to do things with them. I know my son is lonely and I need to spend more time with him, but I like to isolate myself and I can't be bothered to be with him really. I may be playing with him but then I get a flashback and I am not capable of being with him anymore, being present. I am very unhappy about this myself. I wish I could be more present as a father, but it is beyond my ability.*

Even though the couple describe themselves as feeling hopeless and depressed, they have chosen to have another baby, which could be seen as a sign of hope. Fatemeh's feelings of love for her son and husband are an act of resilience as well as her desire to get better someday. Mahdi is being resilient by continuing his political activities in England, even if he speaks of not feeling hopeful about the future.

Fatemeh spoke with expectation about her pregnancy and about how she feels secure in her marriage. She spoke with warmth about her husband and her son and the support she gets from her husband.

> *My husband and I are very kind to each other, very loving. I think this gives me strength to go on. Our son gives us so much love, and I know this baby will too. My husband spends hours reassuring our son, talking to him, comforting him; he talks to him about our future here, together.*

Fatemeh, despite having said earlier that she has little hope of feeling better, showed me she has hopes of getting better, of feeling happy again:

> *I just hope I will start to feel better; I hope. Do you think I will get better someday? I need time to heal. My son is recovering fast. He can sleep better*

now, and I can see he is moving on and putting the past behind him, even if he still has anxiety about certain things, but I can't seem to be able to forget the past.

Mahdi, however, did not speak of hope for the future, not even joy over his wife's pregnancy: '*It doesn't really give me any hope for the future because I don't believe in the future for me because I want to have peace and I'm not sure I will ever find it.*'
Tina is very aware of the effects of the past adverse experiences on her relationship with her husband and her sons.

Because of what happened to me, I cannot be intimate with my husband. Even my son, who is growing a bit of a beard now, when he hasn't shaved and he wants to kiss me, I cannot stand it, it reminds me too much . . . [because the sheikh hadn't shaved either]. I have been so badly damaged by a man, and now my own husband is someone I cannot look up to, so that makes things worse. I don't even sleep in the same room with my husband, let alone have any form of physical contact. I still have feelings for him even if I question my feelings sometimes and wonder if they are real or if I am fooling myself.

You know, I have changed so much; I am a completely different person to the one I used to be, so my husband doesn't know me anymore. We were extremely close, but unfortunately that has all gone; we are now so far apart mentally and emotionally, there is an enormous gap between us. My husband can see how anxious I am all the time, how unhappy I am with our current way of living, our situation. We both agree that a relationship should be full of love and tenderness towards each other, only then can you be intimate. He can see we don't have that at all anymore. He does get irritated sometimes if he, for example, wants to sit close to me on the sofa, and even then, I run away. He gets irritated and says, 'what's wrong, did I give you an electric shock?' He does get irritated at these things.

Tina also spoke clearly about her changed relationship with her sons and cried a lot because it was painful for her to admit how much the traumatic experiences have affected her family.

When the boys are home, they may be talking and laughing with their father, having a good time, but it irritates me, and I lose my temper even then. I can often get rude, tell them to shut up and things like that. Then I think afterwards 'my God, it's as if you don't even want to see your children's happiness'. I have no patience (with the boys) and can't really be bothered with them; I can't spend time with them like I used to. I am very angry with myself over this and want to be the kind of mother I used to be, but I can't. I always used to find them the best schools, for example, I used to be involved in their education. But now I just feel lost, and I feel God likes me anyway because the way I am my kids shouldn't be doing well in school, but they are okay. My older son is worried about our relationship as a couple. Both boys (my poor darlings), I feel as soon as they see us getting into an argument; they try to distract us and come in between. The boys hate to see me like this; if I have a bit of white hair showing they get upset and want me to be the way I used to be.

Hamed spoke in a matter-of-fact way about his relationship with Tina, as if he had accepted it and could no longer feel hurt or bothered.

All these difficulties have had a terrible effect on our couple relationship. We have no intimate relationship and haven't had since we fled Afghanistan. My wife no longer trusts me or respects me, at all, at all. Whenever I say anything, she attacks me and contradicts me; she belittles me to the extreme in front of our sons. My wife and I just no longer have a relationship, not socially, emotionally, mentally, nothing. We just live under the same roof that's all. We are completely far apart from each other. My wife is constantly looking for a fight; she nags and complains to drive everyone crazy. It's as if she constantly wants to harm me, punish me.

Hamed is aware of his changed position as a father and of how different the family dynamics are from how they used to be before their flight.

Unfortunately, as a father, my sons don't respect me or listen to me at all, at all! Before they used to listen to everything I said; not anymore. . . . They don't trust me anymore either. They don't share any of their worries with me; they no longer count on me as a father. None of them hold any value for me. None of them have any value for me at all! I keep thinking about how to kill myself. I have lost everything, my life, my sister, my wife and my sons. Even my son, my oldest, has no aim in life or joy in life; he hardly goes to college, he hardly goes out; he is also depressed. The problem is that whatever I say to my sons they act as if I don't know anything. Before they thought I knew everything and listened to me, now they almost make fun of the things I say. The constant arguments we have are very harmful to our children, they have had so much to deal with and now as well.

What Hamed and Tina make clear in what they say is the impact of the traumas on at least two generations; the boys seem to be affected and damaged by their past experiences of trauma as well as their current experience of having two absent parents who isolate themselves and cannot bear to talk about their thoughts and emotions. They each hurt in isolation, mother, father, older brother and younger brother. Maybe the boys do not speak in order to protect their fragile parents, or maybe they learnt at an early age that this is the family's dominant belief and script; to not express emotions, other than through explosions of anger or self-harm.

Pooneh was extremely sad and even a little angry when she spoke about her relationship with her husband and the new Siavash whom she did not really know.

These five years completely changed our relationship. The hardships, the stress, the fact that he couldn't work; he lost all confidence in himself. He wasn't even capable of looking for a job. He would ask me to call or to go with him to say, 'my husband is looking for work.' I just couldn't get it and kept asking myself 'why did I marry him? What did I do?' We were both so very depressed; me, for instance, I had come to hate myself because I had put myself in that situation for five long years, that's all I thought about and there was no space to think about our relationship. This all caused me to feel more and more distant from him. Now we never talk, we have nothing to say to each other anymore.

Pooneh spoke about the differences in their ambitions and how this is creating even more tension and bitterness in the couple.

The reason we got leave to remain was because of me but my husband will never admit that to me, never a thank you. He never worked, he was not active like me, he didn't even study English and to this day his English is poor. I am the one who wants him to be someone, and he doesn't seem to care anymore. He is distancing himself from me and our daughter. Even if he sees me talking and laughing with our daughter, he asks us to be quiet. When I talk about my work, he gets jealous and stabs me in the back. I don't want to share anything with him. I know he says he is happy for me, but in his actions I see he is resentful that I am moving on and he isn't. He says that since I am working and successful, I don't have the same respect for him and that even our daughter realises it. But I feel he is happy to always play the victim, it suits him.

Siavash is also clearly aware of the impact of the past on their relationship, and he expresses a lot of self-blame.

It has affected our relationship so much; at first it made us much closer and dependent on each other; we only had each other, and we were constantly talking, discussing. But after a while we started looking at someone to blame and we started to drift apart, and the problems we had in our couple were accentuated. I blame myself and I can feel that my wife also blames me for everything, the hardships. We are not close anymore, the way we used to be, not affectionate towards each other; the relationship we had is no longer there. I just don't feel like laughing anymore, don't feel joy, and haven't felt it for the past seven years. Even when my daughter was born, I was happy, but not fully happy. I was sad that she had to be born in such circumstances; I wanted her to be born in the utmost comfort and safety. Even now, when my daughter is lively and happy, I cannot share it with her.

There seems to be a great deal of blaming in this couple, blaming the other and self-blame. One understanding of it may be that they did not *have* to leave for a political reason or because their lives were in danger. They made a conscious decision together, although it was mostly to meet Siavash's urge and need to leave his family behind to protect himself emotionally.

Pooneh blames her husband for their hardships and resents him for not admitting to her how distressing their experiences have been.

> *During this time, the only thought that went through my head was 'how did we end up here? How did we come to this?' We were living our lives in Iran! All the difficulties, to France, to England, then Canada, now here; what were we thinking? I wanted them to send me back to Iran. Then I would think about 'how come I have become this futile person?' I blamed my husband. I said, 'If you had listened to me then, gone to France and applied for a visa for me as your wife, things would not be like this for me.' He is not the kind of person who can accept his errors; he kept saying the responsibility was both of ours, that we had decided together, not just him, and that I had no right to condemn him. This all caused me to feel more and more distant from him. Shadi, I had no one, no support, not my husband, not my family, no friend, no one. I still don't have any support; if I ever want to talk about those days, my husband will still not accept the situation I was in and how very difficult it was for me. He feels no guilt, no remorse, over making me live through such hardships, and that is so very hard for me. My parents kept blaming me for leaving that way, as a refugee.*

Although Siavash starts talking about himself and his wife as 'we', his manner of speech soon changes and becomes one of self-blame.

> *It's as if we didn't quite realise what we were about to embark on, what we had decided to do. We had decided quickly to leave Iran illegally and hadn't really thought about what we were doing. The only reason Pooneh left Iran was because I insisted that she leave. She was happy and she went through all these difficulties because of me. This reality really tortured me, and I still think that if I hadn't been so selfish, her life would have been much better.*

What is interesting to see is that Siavash does acknowledge all the suffering his wife went through but has not shared this with Pooneh, who still believes that he refuses to accept it. This may be because of a sense of pride whereby Siavash does not want to admit to his wife that he had made a bad decision to leave as refugees, or it may be out of anger and the rift between the couple where giving anything is giving too much.

Akbar spoke more in general about how, according to him, most relationships that started in Afghanistan ended when the couple moved to the West. He did not volunteer to talk about his relationship with Nadia, and, out of respect, I did not ask him directly.

When I was with my partner in Afghanistan, it was a man-domineering society and that was reflected in our relationship. When we came to the West, it was as if there was an earthquake in our relationship, and then it was as if in this society it all went in favour of my partner and we finally separated. As long as we were living in the same environment, there was a balance and the relationship worked. Also, in our society the women's place was very different in the couple and society. In Afghanistan I had a lot of status in the couple relationship as well, but in the Swedish society, I had no power or authority. The women say to themselves 'well here we are both on benefit, we are equally low in society, we do not belong to our husbands, we are equal him and I'. So, the woman does not accept a lot of the things she felt she had to accept before. The man then has a choice of whether he wants to adapt to his new role in the couple or not accept and then that leads to separation.

Nadia, however, wanted to speak about her relationship with Akbar and the effects of the past on their relationship.

Talking about relationships, whether it's friendship or intimate, I feel I have a limit in trusting or giving of myself now. One of the biggest effects of prison was to stop me from expressing emotion. I show little or no emotion with my facial expressions. I still wear a mask even if I have tried to work on myself, but this obviously has an impact on my intimate relationship. Usually, peoples' faces are the mirrors of their souls but certainly not mine. The wrinkles on your face are the map of your emotions and experiences, and mine is almost a blank canvas. I was with my partner [Akbar] for many, many years before I told him about my physical disabilities; I hid them from him for years. I would not communicate with Akbar, not give of myself; I would never really express any wishes, thoughts and especially feelings, and all of these led to the break-up of our relationship, although we remain very good friends. We lived together for 14 years, but I never got to the stage where I could give of me really, take the mask off. I also couldn't have children, although I love children, because of the physical torture I suffered.

Akbar spoke about losing his identity in exile and about how this impacts on any relationship he may engage in.

I was trapped because, even if there was work, I couldn't do it because of my lack of language. I therefore only saw myself as an unimportant and broken person in society. Now I was in a situation where I had to constantly ask others for help for everything; it was so difficult. I had had a high and important position from every aspect before, and all of a sudden I had fallen very low; it's not just feeling useless because you can't speak the language, it's every single aspect; you become like a helpless child again who needs someone to hold their hand, you need to go here, do this, this is the train system, this is that, etc.

In Sweden they had given me a number which was my identity, and to me it meant that I was nobody. Whereas in Sweden the society has much more respect for a human being than in Afghanistan, I didn't feel worth much in myself. I was at a level of '0' and I had to say 'give me money, give me a roof, give me education, give me furniture'. That is why for years I cannot remember laughing. My characteristics had changed, and they are still different to this day; I am no longer the person I used to be, at all, at all. No one cared if you lived or died; you could be upset, and nobody cared.

References

Gil, D.G. (1998), *Confronting Injustice and Oppression: Concepts and Strategies for Social Workers*. New York: Columbia University Press.

Van Wormer, K.S. (2004), *Confronting Oppression, Restoring Justice: From Policy Analysis to Social Action*. Alexandria, VA: Council on Social Work Education.

Watts, R.J., Griffith, D.M. & Abdul-Adil, J. (1999). Sociopolitical Development as an Antidote for Oppression: Theory and Action. *American Journal of Community Psychology*, 27(2): 255–272.

Chapter 4

Differences and Similarities

My participants mentioned many themes which they seem to have experienced in common, despite their different lived experiences. I shall take a closer look at these here.

Temporal Framework

The temporal framework is an important one as the themes of pre-flight, flight and post-flight are significant transitional time frames for the couples. I wanted to get a better understanding of the experiences of trauma which each couple had had, and it soon became clear that their experiences of trauma vary significantly, depending on the time and place in which they occurred. Somehow, most of my participants seemed to feel that the traumas they experienced in their home country were more bearable than on foreign ground where they all felt more helpless. This fits with my experience in working with my patients.

The participants who were politically active in Iraq and Afghanistan (Mahdi, Nadia and Akbar) had most of their traumatic experiences in the home country, and their experiences during flight tended to be less traumatic and long lasting. Despite differences in the couple experiences during the period of post-flight which I have discussed, they all seem to share a same sense of hopelessness, although two of my participants, Pooneh and Nadia, have been able to change their feelings of hopelessness to ones of hope.

The second couple (Tina and Hamed) experienced extreme trauma both before leaving Afghanistan and during their flight to England. The couple was different to my other participants in that although they were not politically active, they had fallen victim to the oppressive system of the Taliban regime. Hamed was not befriending intellectual people because he wanted to turn away from Islam; he liked these men for who they were and for their intellect. '*I had a good friend who was very well read. He was someone I had a lot of respect for; he was a very nice and good man.*' However, because of his association with people from the intellectual section of society, their downhill spiral began when his wife was raped by the Taliban who were put into place to watch Hamed and his activities. Tina and Hamed suffered an accumulation of extreme adverse experiences, which enforced

DOI: 10.4324/9781003310716-5

their sense of unsafeness and vulnerability over a rather long period of time. This had a detrimental impact on their couple relationship, which struggled to remain solid. I shall speak about this further under the theme of silence.

The third couple (Pooneh and Siavash) is very different to the other participants because their lives were never in danger in Iran. The young married couple decided to leave Iran, where Pooneh was happily living a comfortable life, because Siavash felt alienated having lived abroad for so many years. There was a sense, for him, of not being able to 'fit in' in the Iranian society, which was painful as he is Iranian himself. He also felt pressured and criticised by his family and wanted to get away and start anew with his wife. Despite all the harrowing experiences they had, following their decision to leave Iran illegally, Siavash maintained that he had no regrets about his decision.

All my interviewees spoke about feeling depressed during the post-flight period; often the deep sadness was associated with feelings of confusion and even self-blame. '*I know I am safe here and should be fine, but I don't know why I am so sad*' (Fatemeh). They all had this same sense of despair in common where they survived through all the difficulties and trauma in Iraq and Afghanistan and on the way to safety, and yet, once they were settled, the sadness crept into their souls. The men seemed to associate their sadness to a state of lost identity, where they no longer have a sense of meaning in their lives. Although Mahdi and Akbar are continuing their political activity in the UK, they did not seem convinced about the usefulness of this. '*I don't believe in the future because I want to have peace but I'm not sure I will find it*' (Mahdi).

Before I carried out the interviews, I thought that being given refugee status in a foreign country was a significant recognition of the sacrifices made by a political activist and their ethical commitment to a better world. Although Mahdi, Akbar and Nadia had all been given refugee status almost immediately upon their arrival to the UK (and for Akbar to Sweden), they did not seem to feel an inner recognition, as if all their fighting had been to no avail. It seems that this sense of doubt (was it really worth it?) may contribute to their deep sadness.

For other participants, like Fatemeh, Tina and Hamed, it seems that they were in survival mode before reaching 'safety' and that whilst struggling to survive, they programmed themselves to function on a day-to-day basis without allowing themselves to ponder upon their experiences and their state of mind. Once they were given leave to remain, their past difficulties and trauma invaded their minds. This is a very common phenomenon I see in my work with refugees.

I had expected immigrants (forced and voluntary) to have a sense of achievement at overcoming the difficulties and making it to safety and perhaps a better future. What I found was a sense of self-blame, despair, anger and guilt. Only two of my participants (Pooneh and Nadia) felt pleased with their power to resist and overcome their difficulties and to create a good future for themselves in the UK. Even Nadia went through a period of feeling depressed and hopeless before she found hope in her books and realised the power of words and how she could continue her fight for her political and ethical convictions through her writings.

It seems that Pooneh's strong sense of self helped her through the difficulties and encouraged her never to give up on herself and her right to a better future.

One essential difference between forced migrants and volunteer migrants may be that my participants were all forced migrants (except for Siavash and Pooneh) and possibly they cannot feel as if they have achieved anything in reaching safety. They are only able to see what they have lost because their losses are both so over-bearing and were forced upon them. As they did not choose to leave, the anger and bitterness seem to stay with them and turn into desolation and hopelessness. There is also a sense of almost having betrayed those who had to stay behind in the country, and the guilt diminishes any feeling of achievement of the refugee.

Gender and Culture

One of striking features in my work with refugees, and through the interviews with these couples, is the difference in the way the male participants seem to have struggled more in the period of post-flight than the female participants. In the Iranian, Iraqi and Afghani culture, the men tend to have a very important role as the provider for the family and gain status within the family and the respect of their wife and children because they provide for them. A woman's role within the family tends to be a different, but also a very important and central, one; they bring up the children and prepare them for going out into society, they run the household and oversee the family budget and have a great deal of power within the family. The father would usually only get more involved in the children's education and upbringing at the request of the mother.

The male participants all spoke about having lost their status and place in society and therefore in the family. In Iranian culture, the professional identity of the man tends to inform the identity of the rest of the family; a doctor's wife is called 'lady doctor', an engineer's wife is called 'lady engineer' and so forth. My male participants share a feeling of uselessness because they are unable to find their place in society and within their family structure. They seem to be holding on to their past identity, and the more they hold on to their past, the less they are able to adapt to their new life and status. I believe this is because they were *forced* to migrate and to leave their established identities behind; as it was not their choice, they seem to not be able to mourn who they were before they were compelled to leave. Some had professional identities which gave them status, such as Hamed, and others had a political identity which gave them power, such as Akbar. Even if Akbar and Mahdi hold on to their past identity by continuing to be politically active, they have clearly lost a substantial part of who they were because they are no longer a person whom others look up to, come to for advice and really count on.

The men I interviewed seem to be holding on to their right to feel sorry for themselves and for their fate, and although understandable, this prevents them from moving forward. If they were able to go through a bereavement period where their past could be recognised and their earlier identities acknowledged, this may help them to move on to the present and possibly the future.

The female participants have all shown a remarkable capacity to adapt to their situation post-flight. Although Fatemeh speaks of her deep sadness, she can still carry hope for the family and is pregnant, which seems to show a sense of seeing the future as positive. Fatemeh clearly stated how she is having a baby to make sure their son is not alone; she is doing it for her son and to give hope to her husband. Pooneh managed to get a very good job as soon as she received leave to remain. She continues to be positive about her present and future situation in bringing up their daughter, making sure she goes to a good school, that they live in a nice area and that she rebuilds their family structure by supporting her husband to succeed in his studies: '*I am the one who keeps pushing him to do things, I push him to study, I help him every night with his homework, translating things for him. I am the one who wants him to be someone.*'

Tina has also shown a sense of reality and not just stayed in the past in that she has taken her children to see a therapist; she has also gone with them to a family therapist. She constantly holds her sons in mind, never forgetting her role as a mother, even if she is less able to do the housework. There is a sense of bereavement in her in that Tina realises that she is no longer able to be the mother she was in Afghanistan, but the way she spoke about the past did not give me the sense that she is stuck in the past, unlike her husband.

Nadia could be mourning the fact that she can no longer have children because of the violence her body has been subjected to, but instead she has decided to 'give birth' to her books. She has faced every challenge with pragmatism and has refused to be defeated. Although Akbar has also managed to adapt well in British society and to build a place for himself, he still feels unsatisfied: '*Even if I feel I have pulled myself out of a big dark hole, I still don't feel that I have achieved much.*' This statement shows how Akbar feels he has not accomplished much compared to what he felt he attained in his political activities in Afghanistan, demonstrating how not mourning the past hinders him from moving forward.

I believe that part of the reason why the female participants have managed to show more resilience is that their fundamental roles as mothers and wives have not changed in the UK. On the contrary, what has changed for all of them is that they can no longer adopt the identity of their husbands, as the husbands have no particular identity here, besides being refugees. Maybe this has urged women like Pooneh to create their own identity more quickly and motivated Tina to get well enough to be able to learn English fast and do something with her life again professionally.

Persian mythology has many important and powerful female figures, and Iranians are brought up bathed in this mythology. The way women are portrayed in Persian mythology influences in turn how women are seen in society. Women are portrayed as being extremely strong minded and resilient mother figures who would show ultimate sacrifice for the benefit of their families. Examples of these extraordinary women are in the famous Persian poet Ferdowsi's 'Shahnameh', which means 'Letters to the King'. The myth tells us about Faranak, who saves her son, Fereidoon, from a giant called Zahaak. Another legendary female figure is Poorandokht, who is a queen and to help create peace with the Romans, takes away the cross on which Jesus was crucified, from Khosroh and Parviz (two men in power in Persia) and gives it back to the Romans. Although the mythology is not as pervasive in Afghanistan, because it is written in Farsi, many Afghanis are aware of the various stories in the 'Shahnameh' and of other Persian mythology.

Returning to the stories of the female participants, I can see how this sense of a mother's sacrifice and resilience spoken about throughout history is particularly evident in Tina's interview. When Tina is being kidnapped and taken in a car to her dark and terrifying destiny, she shows extreme courage in that she tries to mentally prepare for the interrogation she imagines awaits her. '*I was thinking concentrate and think about the kind of answers you are going to give when they ask you questions about the intellectuals.*' It seems that what helped Tina to be so strong at this point was her desire to protect her husband; she felt that if she gave different answers to the questions than those her husband had given during his interrogation; they would arrest him again. When Tina arrives home very late after her ordeal, she continues to show resilience by 'going into her mother role' and making sure her sons are not aware of what has happened to their mother. The desire to hide the truth continues to give Tina the strength to be steadfast as she goes into work the next day, determined that her husband should not suspect that something is wrong. Once again Tina's aim to protect her family helps her to be stalwart.

Immediately upon realising that the threat of the Taliban to her and her family is imminent and that no amount of hiding the truth is going to protect her family or herself, Tina becomes physically resistant to the Taliban and fights back.

Hamed's sister is also a great example of a strong and resilient woman. She showed immense courage and strength when she dispersed the papers she had taken from Hamed's home into the river so that the Taliban could not get their hands on them. In doing so she must have known that she was putting her own life at risk, as she tried to save her brother's life.

Another case of ultimate resilience to protect her loved ones is Fatemeh. Fatemeh's love and respect for her husband allowed her to show resistance and not divulge his whereabouts. She was also able to stand up to the pressure her brothers were putting on her to separate from Mahdi, for the same reasons. Fatemeh's role as a protective and caring mother, and her determination to keep their son safe, gave her strength to resist the torturous interrogations by the Iraqi Secret Service.

The women I interviewed have never forgotten their love and tenderness towards their children and have held their husbands and close family members in mind during extremely difficult times. They have continued to try and create a safe atmosphere for their loved ones through all their trauma and have stayed strong in all three phases of their life changes.

A famous Persian poet, Rumi, says: 'Woman is a ray of God. She is not that earthly beloved: she is creative, not created.'

Silence

When I started the interviews, I expected to discover a measure of conflict in the couple relationships, possibly because of the sometimes uncontrollable anger I had seen in my patients who suffered from post-traumatic stress disorder (PTSD). What I found, instead, was silence. There seems to be different causes for and functions of silence: one of the reasons for the non-communication seems to be self-blame and therefore shame. Hand in hand with this is blaming the other partner. This is very evident in Pooneh and Siavash's relationship, where Pooneh blames her husband and his decision to leave Iran and for all their subsequent adverse experiences. She expects to have some recognition from her husband for the pain and suffering she went through, and yet Siavash, although he did not stop blaming himself during his interview with me, has never once spoken about their past difficulties with his wife. It seemed to me that he could not bear to recognise how much his decision had changed his wife's comfortable and safe life to living a life of uncertainty, fear and psychological torture for many years. Siavash therefore remains silent and refuses to speak about the past, almost blaming his wife for being strong enough to make a future for their family in the UK while he continues to struggle. Pooneh, on the other hand has decided to not confront her husband's silence because she is moving forward and feels that speaking about the past is not going to be helpful, especially as she feels so much anger and resentment inside of her. The silence has therefore created a rift in the couple who were once so close.

In Tina and Hamed's couple relationship, silence and secrecy has played a protective role in that Tina has tried to protect her husband and family by withholding the truth about the rape, knowing that if her husband knew, he would try to go after the perpetrator and by doing so, put the family at more risk. It has also helped Tina to avoid a sense of judgement by her husband, who, she says, would always see her differently if he knew she had been raped. The secrecy has, however, also played a destructive role in that it has created a significant rift in the couple where the secret is so big and omnipresent that any communication seems either dangerous or futile. The secrecy has also caused deceit, where Hamed is left believing they had to leave Afghanistan because of his friendship with more intellectual men and he is self-blaming. However, were he to know that the man who was put in his restaurant because of his intellectual friends has raped his wife, he may not be able to forgive himself. The silence does not just exist in the couple relationship; even their sons have decided to remain silent about the past. They seem to have adopted the family script that things should not be spoken about as this may cause more pain. They are therefore left to deal with the hurt and trauma on their own, where they do not even dare to share with a professional, despite the support and encouragement of their mother. They have clearly understood the message that communicating is too risky. Paradoxically, Tina and Hamed each expressed relief and gratitude for having been given the opportunity to talk to me. They said they felt safe to tell me everything they felt they wanted to, knowing that it would not be shared with the other partner and knowing that they would not have to see me again.

In Fatemeh and Mahdi's relationship, both remain silent about their feelings of despair, and neither has spoken to the other about what they each went through before they came to the UK separately. Mahdi has not told Fatemeh about the amount of torture he suffered in prison, and Fatemeh has never told him about her nomadic life with their son, always in hiding and under pressure. They each want to protect the other from being more distressed and feeling guilt, and yet, as each can see the suffering of the other, the silence weighs heavily in the house, and their son tries to create life and to distract and protect his parents. Fatemeh told me she cannot feel real joy over her pregnancy but can see how happy it makes her husband, and Mahdi spoke of not feeling any joy but knowing that his wife was happy over her coming baby. Although it may seem that they are being deceitful to each other, in this couple, unlike other participants, I did not have the sense that they were living separate lives; I felt how much they still love and care for each other and despite the silence, there was a clear sense of togetherness and warmth in the couple and the family. I think this may be because Fatemeh married Mahdi knowing he was politically active and accepted the life they would lead from the start. Somehow, therefore, the traumas they experienced were expected.

Although Nadia and Akbar were both politically active and openly so, they each remained silent about their harrowing experiences. Akbar never shared his fear of mosques and Islam with Nadia, and she remained stone faced and silent about her eight years in prison. In this couple, it does not seem to be a silence to protect the other, as much as to protect oneself and one's integrity. Although Nadia is disabled and was constantly having to go to the hospital for various appointments, she remained silent about her health problems and never once shared her aches and pains with her partner. In the end, the silence and secrecy created so much distance between them that they decided they were no longer a real couple, just two individuals sharing the same flat.

I have come to understand that having worked with refugee families for so many years, I was never aware of the destructive silence which creates a situation in which the couple lives side by side and yet so far from each other. They seem to be living on separate islands with a cold and dangerous sea between them. The effect of this on the children who suffer not only from their past traumas but also from their present situation seems to be significant. Even though conflict can be unhealthy for a family, it still means communication, and I suppose, to me, as long as there is communication there is hope. The silence I have discovered is threatening because it seems that there are no bridges between these islands, not even broken, wobbly ones; there therefore seems to be less hope. This is where therapeutic help becomes essential, where the therapist needs to help the family members to build bridges. I shall be talking more about my work with refugees later in the book. Thinking about it as I write my thoughts now, I realise that in my family we never spoke about the things we had had to leave behind either. We never mourned our loss as a family; each of us dealt with our pain and loss separately. We did, however always remain close as a family and my parents were resilient and positive, and we knew we could count on them. They did not allow the difficulties to break them as individuals, as a couple or as parents. I suppose what was different in my situation is that we were not refugees and we left Iran knowing my father had a job in Sweden.

I healed through writing about my feelings of despair. I remember sharing my writings with my mother and we would cry together, remembering the past, remembering our country, remembering our life together when we had friends and family around us . . . Perhaps trauma and loss silences us because it is too hard to bear, and even harder to express; perhaps my participants have numbed their feelings to have the strength to live in the present, pretending the past never happened.

Regarding the silence, I notice how it can also stop my participants and the families I work with from befriending other people from their home countries. The shame refugees can feel about their experiences of trauma in all three stages of their flight, seems to force them into silence and a mistrust of others, even if these others are their fellow compatriots who have probably been through similar ordeals to their own. This mistrust leads to them being even more isolated and unsupported, and healing is therefore further delayed.

All my participants, as well as the refugees I work with, speak of their isolation, of not having the support of friends and family here and how much the solitude weighs on them. In Iran, Afghanistan and the Arab countries, individuals and families tend to be surrounded by family, friends and neighbours; everybody is involved in everybody's life. Even on the street, if a parent tells off their child and smacks them, passers-by get involved and ask the parent to be gentle and try to understand what the problem is! There is no such thing as personal space in our culture and we are brought up surrounded by 'others', whether these others are family, friends or strangers. Perhaps this entourage of care and support helps refugees to be more resilient in their home country, and when they are on their own, without even the support of each other in the couple relationship, the loneliness is a constant reminder of their loss and all the symbolic things they could not bring in their suitcases.

I am also aware of how, in my culture, things tend to not be said and spoken about. In Iran we tend to believe that talking about difficult memories or situations makes things worse and hurts too much. The death of a family member is, for example, hidden from those who live abroad so as not to hurt their feelings, and bad news is lied about to protect. I have noticed this same tendency in my Afghani, Kurdish and Arab families.

I remember that my healing took many years; I have shared one of my writings (Addendum 2). It is something I wrote two years after I had left Iran, yet if I had not written the date on which I wrote this, I would not have thought that it was two years after I had left everything; it reads as if I have only just left my past life. This is similar to the experience I had in my interviews and in my work with refugees, where participants had all spoken in the present tense when speaking of the past, as if when loss and trauma happen, the sense of time gets lost and confusion takes over. I also notice that, in my writing, I am telling myself to lock away my memories and not acknowledge the loss; I had clearly also understood the family script of not mourning the past and just moving on to the present.

One other thing which I have noticed about my participants is that each and every one of them has had the capacity and the strength to maintain his/her/ their sense of humanity, generosity, kindness and caring for the other. They each showed exceptional hospitality and mindfulness towards me during the interviews, and I felt humbled by their humanity towards me. The hardships have not hardened them as human beings, and this gives me a great sense of hope and of wanting to be one with them. I do not want to take a distance or a meta position as 'the interviewer'; I want to be one with them and embrace their lived experiences and learn from their humility and kindness. In my therapeutic work with my refugee clients, I take the same position of being with them, alongside them and a reassuring presence.

References

Ferdowsi c 977–1010CE. *Shahnameh.*
Rumi Mathnawi I, 2421–2437 (13th century Iranian Poet), *Loves Ripening.*

Chapter 5

Seeking Therapeutic Help and Cross-Cultural Therapy

To get a better understanding of refugees' experiences of the therapeutic help they have received in England as well as how to improve therapeutic services for refugees, I not only interviewed the four couples about their experiences and wishes, I also interviewed two Farsi-speaking therapists (from charity organisations) who work with Farsi-speaking refugees from Afghanistan, Iran and parts of Kurdistan, Marjan and Arash, as well as an English family therapist, Sophie, who has extensive experience working with refugees in the National Health Service (NHS). By doing this I tried to get the perspective of the service users as well as the professional caregivers and looked at the emerging themes for both groups.

The Importance of Language

Interpreters

Although my English colleague, Sophie, spoke about the positives of working with an interpreter, my other participants emphasised the importance of speaking the same language.

According to Sophie, it can be valuable to work with an interpreter because a good interpreter can act as a consultant and explain cultural practices. The male Farsi-speaking counsellor I interviewed, Arash, spoke about an Afghani woman he once worked with who was very well educated and came from a well-off family; her husband was a doctor in Afghanistan. According to Arash, as she was speaking about her children, she said '*I have two children and a girl*'. Arash spent the rest of the session challenging this statement and wondering about the place of a girl in the Afghani family and culture, even in a well-educated family such as theirs. According to Arash, this session enabled the family to reconsider their family dynamics. They even had discussions about girls' names in Afghanistan which show their place in society, names such as 'Kaafi', which means 'enough', and what the significance of this must be for the girl. I asked Arash whether he thought a non-Farsi-speaking therapist could have challenged the family's position towards gender in the same way, and he said that an interpreter would never have interpreted such a thing to 'keep face'. An interpreter would have said 'I

DOI: 10.4324/9781003310716-6

have two sons and a daughter' and then as a therapist you would have not had a real understanding of the family dynamics. I am actually not certain that in any case the family would have accepted a challenge from a 'foreign' therapist because the Afghani family may have felt judged by an occidental therapist.

Regarding service users' perspectives, Mahdi, who is Iraqi, said it was important to him to see a therapist who speaks his language. '*I didn't like seeing a therapist with an interpreter because the interpreter can never say what I am saying, the way I am saying it. I much preferred to speak my own language.*' Tina was also very clear about the importance of language in therapy:

> I am completely against going to see an English therapist if you are foreign. When the cultures are so different, the person cannot understand you; also, you must speak through an interpreter, and often I could hear that they weren't translating what I had said. Especially in therapy you want the therapist to get what you are feeling! This feeling cannot be told through an interpreter, never in a lifetime. And if the therapist is English, even less chance of them getting what you're feeling because our cultures are so different.

Hamed also expressed how being able to speak the same language as his therapist was important to him:

> I want to go to the Medical Foundation because I know they have Farsi-speaking therapists there who are used to working with Afghanis who have had the same experiences as me. I need to see someone like you who can understand my language and me, ME!

The participants seem to all agree that working with a therapist who speaks your language is essential and makes a great difference in the way you can share your thoughts and emotions. Although Sophie sees the interpreter as assisting her in better understanding certain aspects of the culture, the Farsi-speaking counsellor pointed out the limitations of working through an interpreter and how they often filter what is translated. I myself have many times observed how interpreters change translations to 'keep face'. One example is when I went to accompany one of my patients to court, where she had to explain why she was unable to work because of her mental state. Every time the judge asked questions such as 'Can you walk down the street and go on a bus by yourself?' or 'Do you take a shower every other day?' my patient would answer 'No' because she was unable to do these simple things. The interpreter would always translate these 'No's as 'Mostly I can but not always.' In the end I had to ask the judge for permission to speak and told her that the interpreter was changing what the patient was saying, which was hindering the judge's correct assessment of the situation. When questioned about this, the interpreter admitted that he found it shameful to say his fellow co-patriate did not shower every day and could not be more independent (which are all signs of depression and PTSD). In doing my interviews I spoke in Farsi except for the interview with the Iraqi couple, but because I used an interpreter I had worked with for many years, I felt comfortable and knew that I could trust her to say what the couple were saying verbatim because she knew my way of working as well.

Importance of Cultural Knowledge

Another theme which came up in all my participants' accounts was the importance of the therapist's awareness of the culture of the client. This is something all the refugees I work with say they appreciate in working with me, that I understand their culture and can allow myself to challenge certain cultural beliefs without them feeling judged by me.

The counsellors were able to give examples of how when the counsellor and family come from different cultures it can impact on the therapeutic work. Of course, we must never take for granted that we 'know' the person's culture just because we are from the same country because even within the country the culture may vary; however, when my patients from Middle Eastern counties say to me 'you understand what I mean' I feel I do, and if I do not understand, this to me is a generous invitation from the patient to ask more about their culture and to be curious.

'Otherising'

This theme was evident in what the Farsi-speaking counsellors were telling me and relates to refugees 'otherising' professionals as those who will not be able to understand. This becomes clear in Marjan's account:

> One thing I have noticed is that even before seeing an English-speaking therapist they [Farsi-speaking clients] have their guard up. They already 'know' that the therapist will not be able to understand them or help them. The patients I see always say 'how can they [English therapist] understand us when they have such a different culture?' So, we, as foreigners, have prejudices just as the English-speaking therapists have prejudices about us, and these prejudices on both sides create resistance. The refugees do therefore not open up or talk freely, and they always hide things about their lives, past or present. There is also a sense that we should not let the English know about everything, to not show ourselves. It is so important in our culture to not lose face in front of others, especially if they are foreigners!!

What Arash says reinforces this sense of 'us' versus 'them':

> Iran, Kurdistan and Afghanistan are countries where there have always been many different stressors, both political and historical, which have destabilised and perturbed the whole society. When you look at these, you [Shadi] and I know the effect of these on the people of that country. I think that when Farsi-speaking clients say they are not understood by Western

therapists, they really are not understood, and I see daily examples of it. You need to have knowledge of that particular society and its complexities to understand the different classes and so forth; you may have studied years to be a therapist, but if you don't have this knowledge, you just cannot help. It's like teaching you gardening, but only gardening in a square garden, with a garden centre nearby where you can buy all you need; then they ask you to do gardening in the middle of the desert, with nothing. Can you do the same gardening there, or do you have to adapt to that atmosphere? So usually, therapists in the West are white and middle class, do you think they can help people from such different backgrounds and cultures? They don't fit into their gardening pattern!!

The service users also spoke about the importance of feeling understood in their culture and background in a therapeutic relationship and seemed convinced that they could not be understood by therapists from another culture.

Tina was explicit about how important culture is.

I mean the English psychotherapists to me (and I have seen many of them) always say, 'well why don't you tell your husband [about the rape], he will be supportive of you'. This shows me they just don't get it! They are clueless about our culture and what you can and can't say.

Siavash also commented on the difficulty of engaging in therapy with a therapist from another cultural background:

I went to see a therapist once, but I felt she just didn't understand, she was in a dream state, not in my reality, my difficulties. I only went once and felt so misunderstood, it was an English therapist. She just could not get it; she was in another world, very different to mine.

Although Nadia had a good experience of getting therapeutic help, she still said,

Even though the therapist was very nice, I felt there were still language barriers and cultural barriers, even if I felt comfortable with her. Often, I do feel that the therapists here have lived such protected lives compared to the life I've lived that they cannot comprehend my experiences; it is too much for them to take on board, no matter how much they try, they just can't!

Making Presumptions

Marjan spoke about often noticing how her colleagues assume that certain things are cultural when they are not. I have seen this many times in my work in Sweden, France and England, where colleagues have understood certain behaviours as being cultural or culturally accepted when they are not. Similarly, they may misjudge a parent in their parenting when their attitude or actions are culturally appropriate. Arash said:

> *Most families in the West have very different problems to us on the other side of the world. In the West, they have smaller stresses in life, like their child going to school. In a place like Afghanistan, the whole society has been turned upside down and is in pieces; this therapy system would not work there. So, when refugees say 'foreigners don't understand us', they really don't. I was referred a client (an Afghani woman) by an English psychiatrist once because he wondered if she was being honest about her symptoms; he thought she was making up symptoms in order to get leave to remain as a refugee. He explained that the patient spoke of getting panic attacks and yet when the psychiatrist asked her about her past experiences she had not been in detention or had any difficulties in Afghanistan. I spent a long time asking about her everyday life here and her route to school, for example. She said that where she lived, they were doing building work and that every time she saw a crane her heart would sink, and she felt panicked. She said, 'back in Afghanistan, every morning when I came out to walk to school, I would see people hanging from the cranes; that was what they were there for.' When the psychiatrist had asked her why she was traumatised, he only asked if she had been tortured, hit, etc., and she answered 'no', so the psychiatrist thought she was lying about being traumatised. Of course, if you don't know what is going on in Afghanistan you cannot possibly know why she is traumatised. Because of my knowledge about life in Afghanistan, I was able to open the conversation and to get her to talk about what she had seen daily, and she was not ashamed to tell me about it. This woman wanted to stop seeing the psychiatrist because she rightly felt not understood at all and also judged by him.*

When Arash was telling me this, as soon as he said 'cranes' I knew exactly why the woman was traumatised because I know some of the context there.

Sophie also spoke about the importance of knowing the client's culture. She said that she tried to build trust in the therapeutic relationship by talking about the cultural differences between them. I believe this is a helpful way of showing genuine curiosity when trying to build rapport with a client, and to share your own culture is an important part of this.

Amongst the service users, Akbar expressed disappointment with his experience of getting help from a non-Farsi-speaking therapist:

> *The therapist had no understanding of the Afghani society and the transitions we had gone through as a nation, in the family, in society, the invasion, and the war, all the transitions. I could not explain it to her, and she could not be of help to me. No, it was no use. I think therapy can only help if the therapist knows or understands your culture, the place you come from, your societal history, and these things which form you, make you, mould you. Only through*

having this knowledge can the therapist then know which questions to ask in order to help the patient express his thoughts and feelings.

I remember an Iranian patient of mine telling me about an incident which had happened to him which had put him off seeing a European therapist; he had felt uncomfortable with his interpreter and had called his therapist before his next session to let him know this. The therapist said he understood, but at his next session the same interpreter was there, and the therapist wanted my patient to explain to the interpreter why he felt uncomfortable with him so that they could discuss it together. My patient felt extremely uneasy because it is not in our culture to confront people like that. The therapist was insensible, and the patient never went back. To me, this shows how therapists can often transfer their own culture and assumptions onto other cultures. In our culture, we do not speak openly about things, especially if they are negative, and explaining to an interpreter why you do not want him/her/them is extremely uncomfortable for both the client and the interpreter.

The comments my participants made on several occasions about feeling the therapist could not understand them because their background and lived experiences were so far apart, brings me on to the next theme; the theme of the therapist being overwhelmed by what they hear because it is too painful or even hard to believe sometimes, which makes the client feel not believed and unheard. Sophie spoke about this in her interview where she often feels overwhelmed when working with refugees and feels that the literature does not reflect reality and is therefore not helpful. There is a sense of hopelessness in her tone:

I think it's very difficult to talk about hope and resilience, even though I know that it is our job to give that kind of hope, but when there are just so many things happening to the benefits cuts, to people with illnesses being told they have to work, even though we know there aren't any jobs. I find it really difficult because there are so many levels of trauma that working with the family is very complex. Where do you start? I mean in the team we often feel like we are in a fog all the time.

Many times, I have seen professionals doubt that what the refugee is telling them is the truth, as the level of oppression they speak of is alien to a Western therapist in that it just does not exist in the same way in Western countries; it is unimaginable to a Western therapist.

Prejudice

Sophie brought up a very important point about the political context and its implications on the therapeutic relationship:

There is such a huge amount of loss, massive loss, of that way of life. I also think that an added complication is that they are in a host country that invaded their country (Iraq) and actually is the reason they had to leave their country. So, it is very, very complicated and they feel they cannot trust anyone. I think it's complex when you're working systemically because people's reaction to having a refugee from, say, Iraq in this country, and who then criticises this country, brought out strong reactions in the team. Reactions like 'they should be grateful', ' we've given them this this and this'. I was surprised at my colleagues' reactions. I mean when you think refugees get passed around services, I was quite shocked at what is happening behind the scenes. And they would get angry at the man and his family for not being able to reflect the way they wanted him to!! I think there are irritations in working with refugees often because there is a sense of stuck-ness in refugees and refugee families. I mean, in couple work, where do you even start because where they would normally get their strengths from each other, now their relationship is a big source of stress for them instead. I also feel that working with refugee couples is extremely difficult because they each have so many complex needs individually, and there is no point in even trying to involve the children because they always want to protect them, as they say, from what is going on.

I believe that Sophie makes some very important points about the ambiguous feelings Western therapists can have when working with refugees. Because the work is so difficult and demanding and slow, the therapist may feel irritated at the client, and the client is going to be aware of this. Maybe that is why some of my participants also felt they were being doubted and not believed. It is imperative to go at the patient's pace, and with refugees they need to repeat things over and over again and in joint sessions with colleagues I have heard them say to the refugee 'yes, you have told me before'. This is taken as being rude in our culture, and it also shows that the clinician has little understanding of the need the refugee has of being acknowledged in their suffering and being heard in their adverse experiences which they live through on a daily basis. A comment like 'yes you have told me before' just shuts the refugee down and creates a sense of mistrust towards the therapist where the refugee goes into his/her shell.

The service users gave examples of when they felt the counsellor was not able to help because they were either overwhelmed or not trusting of their clients.

Pooneh recounts her experience of having seen a therapist once: '*I never went again because I felt in her attitude that she thought I was lying; I couldn't stand her attitude and never went to see anyone again. I am not willing to be treated as a liar.*'

Hamed, who has tried to commit suicide several times, said:

They always say I am fine, and I feel like I have to justify myself and prove to them that I need help. They don't believe me; all I want is to get empty, to empty myself of everything, but I feel they think I am trying to get benefits. I need to get empty; now that I am talking to you, I feel better, that's what I need, someone to just listen and empathise, to help me get empty of these feelings and sadness.

Tina also spoke about feeling unheard, probably because the therapist felt overwhelmed with her story:

> *I went to see a therapist after having attempted suicide a couple of times, when I was very low, and she said to me 'light a candle and sit and look at it!' Maybe that is the right thing to do for some, but I felt so unheard! To take deep breaths, to light a candle, how is that going to help me now?*

Akbar also spoke of having seen a therapist who was overwhelmed by his story and therefore unable to help:

> *I spoke about my past, but the therapist was overwhelmed with my experiences; it was too much for her. It was too unlike anything she knew, and she could not comprehend and almost believe what I was telling her. She had no idea of the war I had fought or the life I had lived, it was too strange for her. I felt I had to educate her too much in order for her to even be able to listen to me.*

Sophie spoke about her struggle in finding the right tools to work with refugees and their complex needs:

> *I must say that I get frustrated that I cannot find more help in the literature when working with refugees because there seems to be no fit between what is written and the reality. I mean, I have read a lot and all the stuff about adversity-activated resilience; it doesn't fit. I feel that sometimes when you touch on their strengths, refugees feel unheard and emphasise everything that isn't the way it should be. But I feel there is a matter of splitting their realities when you start talking of positive effects. I do think you have to be very careful when working with refugees not to talk so much about positives or strengths when they have been through so much trauma. It just doesn't fit, and it feels disrespectful to what they are going through. I feel it is not witnessing, not hearing, not staying with them in all their suffering to witness. But then I suppose I also wonder how long you witness for; it's like they say in the literature that you witness for so long and then you start challenging, it's just not like that!*

Sophie makes an interesting point, which I have also come across in literature, and I share her thoughts about not wanting to focus too much on the resilience people have for fear of not hearing their distress, and it is a difficult and essential balance to hold in mind.

With all the complexities of refugees' past and present, it would seem even more important to provide continuity of care in order to create a sense of safety and to enable the client and therapist to build a trusting therapeutic relationship, yet all of my participants spoke about being passed around amongst professionals. Many of the refugees I work with and my participants spoke about being confronted with different therapists without being forewarned. They were never really told why the therapist had changed, and they gave up caring in the end and went back even deeper into their shells. The refugees often complain of not being respected enough to be informed about their therapist changing and just being expected to get on with it.

Tina said,

> So, they then sent me to yet another psychologist and actually none of them were helpful. I had so many different psychologists who none of them helped me, they were of no use. The last therapist I worked with was at the refugee therapy centre, and I felt she was helping me, but then the number of sessions were limited and came to an end, and when it stopped I felt it really damaged me. The therapist was Iranian, and what she said made sense; I felt she understood me. I was so very upset when the therapy stopped, in the middle of the therapy, when I was feeling so vulnerable and in need.

Hamed had a similar experience of interrupted and haphazard help:

> The therapists keep changing every six months, which is unhelpful. I used to see a counsellor at a care centre, and I have asked many times to be introduced to the Medical Foundation but have been told they cannot see me. My GP keeps giving me medication because I was feeling very low. But I tried to commit suicide with it three months ago and begged the GP to send me to a therapist. I went to see her for a few sessions, three times in six months, but then the therapist changed. I wanted to see the therapist more often, but she would only give me an appointment every two months. When I saw the therapist had changed, I got upset and said I had to start all over again; he said I didn't need to because it was all in the file, but I cannot trust him or someone new all the time.

Bearing in mind how difficult it is for refugees to build a trusting relationship with a therapist, it seems almost emotionally abusive to keep changing the therapist after a few sessions, or indeed to stop the therapy all together; this causes a great deal of harm to the refugee.

Chapter 6

Thoughts on Engaging and Helping Refugee Families in Therapy

Western psychological health care agencies are finding themselves increasingly concerned with assisting traumatised individuals originating from non-Western cultures. This increased demand has been associated with considerable political, practical and resource issues. Health services have been said to have difficulty in adapting to this need, and deficits in care have been reported in the media. For example, an article in the *Guardian* (Grierson 07.04.2021) carried the title 'Home Office to send more asylum seekers to "unsuitable" Napier barracks'. Indeed, services still struggle to catch up with demand and to modify practices accordingly. However, there also seems to have been an increase in professionals' awareness of these complexities and the need to work differently with refugees and their various backgrounds, trauma and cultures. Published work in the past two decades on trauma and refugees, survivors of war, organised violence, oppression and torture seem to be the fastest-growing client group being written about with respect to clinical models of trauma. However, the inevitable difficulty still remains that no matter how much theory you read, the reality is that working with refugees is complex, emotionally stressful and potentially overwhelming to therapists faced with the degree of suffering and trauma experienced by their clients.

In recent years, family therapy has moved towards a more postmodern and social-constructionist perspective. We are now aware that relationships between people are influenced by certain socio-political contexts, such as gender, race, culture and class. This means that the therapist is no longer seen as someone neutral, but he/she/they is also influenced by his/her/their experiences, which in turn influences the therapeutic relationship and so forth. This is evident in Sophie's recount of how some of her colleagues spoke about their refugee clients needing to be grateful to be in England and therefore having less tolerance and understanding of their slow progress in the therapeutic process.

Having worked in the therapeutic field for so many years, I have come to see how most therapists tend to see themselves as non-judgemental and lacking in bias; however, all humans are coded to see and notice difference and to respond to difference, often with negative emotions, simply because we find difference hard to understand and therefore threatening. If, as therapists, we are in denial of our conscious and unconscious biases, I consider that there is a danger of sabotaging

DOI: 10.4324/9781003310716-7

the therapeutic relationship. We need to understand and accept our own unconscious biases in order to be able to build a therapeutic relationship with the refugee. We therefore need to be constantly curious about our thoughts and feelings, to be open about these in supervision and when talking to colleagues.

Working cross-culturally is very challenging, as the therapist has to try and understand the influences of the family they are working with from a different cultural and religious background and then understand how that impacts him/her/them as a therapist and therefore the therapeutic relationship. There are indeed many complex levels of context which influence the therapeutic relationship, and the therapist needs to have a good understanding of these and his/her/their own resonances in order to be able to create an atmosphere of trust which will be stable throughout the many ups and downs of working with refugees and refugee families. Having regular supervision with a trusted supervisor is essential in unpacking all the different levels in the therapeutic relationship with a refugee who is so different to us in culture, race and religion, to name a few, but who has also suffered unimaginable loss and trauma.

The Complexities of Working with Refugees

Sophie, who has worked with refugees for many years, spoke clearly about feeling overwhelmed by the amount of complexity and need which refugees show. Many of my participants described feeling almost put off by therapy when they felt their therapist could not take in what they were recounting and where they therefore felt disbelieved. Much of the disbelief is based on a lack of knowledge of the society and political and religious context the refugees are fleeing. I was working with an Afghani man once who had suffered unbearable trauma when his wife had been raped by two Taliban men in front of him. It had all started when they had gone on a family holiday; their son had been arrested at a party and had been taken to the local police station because parties are forbidden. His son had been given 20 beatings of a whip, and the father (my client) had protested, saying they had no right to treat his son that way. The Taliban men had therefore decided to teach him a lesson and had raped his wife in front of him to show just how much rights they have in the Taliban regime. When my client had recounted his horrendous experience to a young colleague of mine, my colleague came to see me to say he felt the man was making the story up because it sounded unrealistic that things would escalate so quickly and he just found it hard to believe. I had to explain to my colleague that these are common everyday experiences in Afghanistan, that there are no rules except for the ones the Taliban make and that one is at their mercy. I felt my colleague even doubted *my* word and it felt extremely uncomfortable. I therefore asked to work with the man myself, as I did not want him to feel disbelieved in his ordeal.

Alayarian (2007) also speaks about the challenges of working with clients with traumatic stories. She says that if we, as therapists, have had experiences similar to our clients, yet have not worked through them, we are at risk of projecting our issues onto them in countertransference. If we have not shared similar experiences, we cannot even comprehend the unspeakable things we hear, and we find it overwhelming to deal with. I think a way of becoming more acquainted with refugees' experiences is simply by working with them because over time the practitioner will come to understand more and more about the refugees' stories and thereby be less overwhelmed. On the other hand, the refugee may see the therapist as a delicate individual and may therefore withhold information about their experiences for fear of upsetting the therapist. Furthermore, if the therapist is of the host country, the patient may think the therapist has no idea of his/her/their experience and may not want to have to tell his/her/their story to someone with very little knowledge of their social and political background. This is very evident from Akbar and Tina's interviews where Akbar clearly felt he had to first educate the therapist about his background before she could start to comprehend his narrative and where Tina felt unheard because the advice the therapists gave her went against her core cultural beliefs.

I agree with Papadopoulos (2001) that when working with refugees from a systemic perspective, we need to bear in mind two perspectives, one being the essentialist perspective, which reminds us that refugees have had a multiplicity of losses and have been exposed to many painful situations. This perspective helps us to remember that regardless of whether refugees have psychological needs, all refugees have financial, medical, educational, social and numerous other needs which need to be thought about. The other perspective Papadopoulos speaks about is a constructivist perspective, which focuses on the ways refugees define themselves, their needs and their experiences in the context of wider socio-political constructs. Papadopoulos (2001) goes on to say that by positioning ourselves so that we are aware of the pain and vulnerability, as well as the resilience of the individual, family or group, we can begin to work in ways which can empower the survivors of trauma.

Although none of my participants spoke about wanting their therapist to help them with practical and financial needs, my personal experience of working with refugees is that I have to play the role of their advocate in many ways, whether it is speaking to the Home Office, Housing or Social Services. This seems to be a natural part of the therapeutic relationship and helps the refugee to heal by walking alongside them in their everyday ordeals as well as bearing witness to both their sufferings and their strengths. I remember going with a refugee father to a job centre to explain why he could not be looking for work because he was emotionally unable to do so and to explain that he was in therapy with me. The man I was speaking to was, of course, focusing on doing his job, which was to try to get my client to sign up for job interviews, and no matter how much I explained, the employee would not understand and lift the pressure off of my client. I found myself feeling utterly helpless faced with the bureaucracy of the system and how inhumane it all was, and I began to raise my voice in rage at the injustice of the situation where, with every letter my client received from the job centre, he was re-traumatised and fearful. I asked to speak to the manager, and at that point my client gently put his hand on my arm and whispered, 'it's okay, don't get so upset.' When we left the job centre, he thanked me and said that he felt he had had more of a voice through me (even though no one really heard us). This is a refugee's daily ordeal, and to share it with them is part of building the therapeutic alliance and the trust in the therapeutic relationship.

The Importance of Language

All of my participants spoke about the importance of being able to speak the same language as the therapist and, in my experience, language and culture go hand in hand because understanding the client's language is also about understanding the nuances in the language and the meanings these give to lived experiences.

Writing on Iran, Beeman (1976, 1986) introduces two types of communicative system, one aimed at unequivocal direct communication in everyday dealings, and a second with the opposite aim of multiple interpretations and indirect communication. To Western observers directed by their culture and training to think in unambiguous terms, the multiple criteria involved in the Iranian form of communication may leave an impression of uncertainty and even mistrust in social relations. I believe that is why I have often heard my colleagues say that they are unsure of the honesty and authenticity of their Farsi-speaking clients. The clients, in turn, sense this mistrust and feel unheard and judged, as recounted by my participants and clients. According-ing to Beeman, only an outsider would press for a single truth, whereas insiders know that there are many more than one reason for the need to protect appearances and keep face. Systemic therapists would always look for various explanations for a particular pattern of behaviour and would not restrict themselves to a single truth.

Working with Interpreters

This brings up the issue of having to work with interpreters, which has both advantages and disadvantages. It is true that the interpreter can act as the cultural mediator in the triadic relationship between therapist, client and interpreter, but in my experience the relationship with the interpreter can be a very complex one. Often my clients have told me that they stopped seeing their therapist because they refused to say things in the presence of the interpreter, as they did not want to lose face, but also because they did not trust that the interpreter would not spread their story amongst the community. I have, unfortunately, seen how one Iraqi Kurdish interpreter had heard in a doctor consultation where she was translating that a young girl I was working with had an STD and she told the girl's father. Luckily I immediately heard about it from other Iraqi Kurds, and we were able to alert the police and take the girl into protection. Another complexity, especially in the Iranian community, is class; if a family feels that they are from a different class to the interpreter, they will not want to talk in front of them. For a non-Iranian therapist, trying to understand the class system in Iran would take several years because it is not about financial comfort, it is a much more convoluted system.

Ahlberg (2007) has written that there are said to be few societies that take the obligations of status as seriously as the Iranian society does. The Farsi language itself contains a number of stylistic devices to help individuals to communicate to each other such aspects of relationships. Ahlberg goes on to say that interpreters will not explain the symbolic functions of these language subtleties, which in her view are essential in building rapport in the therapeutic relationship. I do not completely agree with this because these rules are only important amongst Iranians themselves; non-Iranians are not expected to understand or respect our ways in the same way. For example, when I see my Farsi-speaking patients, we spend a long time saying hello, an even longer time saying good-bye and almost an endless time inviting the other to leave the room first so that one never has one's back to the other. These are expected of me as an Iranian therapist, but if an English therapist went in front of an Iranian family and entered the therapy room first, the family would not think twice about it. Ideally it would be important that the interpreter translate not only the words but also the emotional meaning of what is said; however, the translation of the full texture of meaning from one language to another requires great skill on the part of the interpreter. I think it is important to acknowledge that sometimes it may be impossible to translate the various layers of meaning and language. One of my colleagues, Dr Eia Asen, taught me to seat the interpreter behind the client so that the therapist and client can be face to face without having the interpreter sit in sight so that you almost forget they are there. This positioning also enables the non-verbal communication between the client and the therapist to be present.

The Importance of Cultural Knowledge

Using Insider Help

Bowen (1978) asserts that the therapist is a 'cultural broker'. Although this is an excellent and welcome idea, it is important to appreciate that, in the case of working with refugee families, this is not always an easy idea to put into practice. To work therapeutically with refugee families can have many complications; these include lack of sufficient knowledge of the refugee families' culture and unique situation as well as the many conflicting positions and perceptions therapists are faced with in relation to these families. In addition, pressures to assist families in their everyday difficulties increase the complexity of therapists' roles. Furthermore, therapists need to be mindful of the refugee families' interrelationships with their environment, and this is difficult to do on their own.

Voulgaridou, Papadopoulos and Tomaras (2006) coordinated a Greek Council for Refugees (GCR) family therapy team which introduced the use of a therapist helper who could be a family member; a member of the wider clan, community or social group of the clients; or a trusted family friend. This person, by assuming the role of a special cultural therapeutic mediator (CTM) (and in close collaboration with the therapists), has the potential to bring about change in the family's construction of the presenting problems and of transforming family members from a closed system within an intra-familial framework which had reached an impasse, to an open system of a meaningful contextual construction. According to Voulgaridou, Papadopoulos and Tomaras (2006), by introducing and collaborating with a CTM, therapists have access to a wider spectrum of the refugee's experiences, beyond the usual focus on either trauma or acculturation. Moreover, by using CTMs, it is easier to access and understand the pre-migrant experiences of the refugee families, as CTMs would share that world with them. A CTM is 'one of them' and, at the same time, functions as a kind of advocate for the refugee family.

Although I agree with this, I must also say that in my experience using a CTM, which in my work is usually an interpreter, who is also used to giving advice on culture, has its own limitations. I have often seen how interpreters will not translate things which they feel is embarrassing, or they will change what the client is saying to 'keep face'. This is also evident from my interview with Arash, who said an interpreter would not have translated what his Afghani client had said as 'I have two children and a girl' but would have just translated it as 'I have three children.' The advantages of using a CTM, as opposed to an interpreter, would be, in my opinion, that they would be a close friend or family member whom the family would have chosen themselves so the barrier of having to say things in front of a stranger the family doesn't trust would not be there.

It is a common phenomenon for refugees to bring along uninvited persons to their psychotherapy sessions. Papadopoulos and Hulme (2002), who studied this phenomenon, called such persons 'transient familiar others'. By conceptualising the position, role and function of CTMs, Voulgaridou attempted to produce what refugees tend to do on their own by bringing along such transient familiar others. Careful attention should be paid to who the client is comfortable with including in sessions while also preserving traditional family roles in the process. In my experience, the client has never wanted to include anyone, family or friend, in the therapy sessions at the beginning of therapy due to feelings of shame and possibly guilt. However, I have often been able to include the spouse and often the children in sessions once trust has been established and a great amount of work has already taken place with the client, allowing them to feel less vulnerable and more contained by me.

Another scheme which has also been used by the GCR team includes therapeutic meetings with wider systems. These may include two or even three families with their own networks and with two or more therapists along with their CTMs. This multi-family and multi-systemic scheme is closer to the concept of natural networks. This approach seemed to be more effective, especially in very stressful situations, such as families with serious illnesses, significant losses and so on. Such schemes generate similar effects to the ones discussed by Papadopoulos (1999) with reference to 'storied communities' and Woodcock (1995) with reference to 'healing rituals'. In my workplace, we also work a great deal with multi-families, and it is always a very efficient way to work where families gain strengths from each other and make important connections, which often helps them out of their isolation. Careful attention needs to be paid, though, to each family's and family members' needs and vulnerabilities in order to create a safe place for them.

Defining Mental Illness in Different Cultures

Culture can influence mental illness by defining the normal and abnormal, by influencing clinical presentation and by determining help-seeking behaviours. Mental illness may not be an acceptable form of presentation in some cultures and may therefore present as psychosomatic symptoms, with non-specific body pains, headaches, dizziness and weakness. This reflects both culturally defined modes of help seeking and their view of appropriate medical presentation. Most of the refugees I have worked with over the years spend their first time in therapy describing their psychosomatic symptoms, and this is an important part of the engagement process where if they can feel heard and taken seriously in their physical suffering, they can then begin to open up more about their emotional and psychological traumas. The refugee's cultural background is likely to determine whether, for example, depression is expressed in psychological and emotional terms or in physical terms.

Ahlberg (2007) refers to the concept of 'Parsities' ('Persian syndrome') which is a term used by frustrated health care professionals in describing their Farsi-speaking patients who often arrive in therapy expecting treatment that is different to what is on offer, such as a request for treatment of a somatic complaint or advice on problems regarding social welfare. This is something I have seen in my Middle Eastern clients.

Owusu-Bempah (2002) emphasises the importance of spiritual well-being in many cultures and the belief in the importance of mystical phenomena in the influence of a person's health and destiny. I know that in the Iranian, Afghani and Kurdish cultures, there is a major place for spiritual beliefs and bad and good spirits which can influence us. Therefore, clinicians practising in multi-ethnic settings must be mindful that beliefs in spirit possession will be involved in some presenting problems of ethnic-minority clients.

Working Cross-Culturally

Effective therapy with families from other cultural backgrounds relies greatly on the therapist's ability to successfully engage the client in the therapy by developing a strong therapeutic alliance. Therapeutic alliance can be defined as the quality and strength of the relationship between client and therapist, developing mutual trust and respect, showing warmth and empathy. As a person's cultural values and belief system are central to all aspects of their lives, displaying empathy, understanding and a genuine interest in a family's culture in the therapy is likely to impact on the effectiveness of therapy and the therapeutic alliance. I once had a colleague who was from South America and said to me with irritation that every client who comes to her from that region assumes she knows their culture and often say to her, 'You know what I mean.' I was surprised at her irritation because to me that sounds like a very generous invitation to ask questions and get to know their culture more. This statement shows that the client wants to trust you as a therapist and is asking you to join them in trying to understand their culture, belief systems and values. Of course, one must never assume to 'know' a culture, but one must always be curious, accepting and respectful of the client's culture.

There is a general belief within the existing literature that therapists need to align themselves with the client's viewpoints and create a safe and containing environment to discuss all aspects of culture-specific material. I believe that there is almost a view that challenging any of the client's beliefs may be seen as being judgemental and non-accepting of difference. But then, I want to ask, how do we enter into a helpful dialogue with our clients if we accept everything they say as 'truth'? How do we attempt to move them forward and help them, for example, to better connect with their young teenager who was brought up here and may have other values than the parents? I worked with a single Afghani mother for over a year, and we had done eye movement desensitisation and reprocessing (EMDR) on her past traumas and had really built a trusting therapeutic relationship. She came to me once crying with despair over the fact that she had found out her 17-year-old daughter had a crush on a boy in her school. She was inconsolable, saying that she was going to send her daughter back home, regardless of the consequences, and she kept speaking of the shame she felt. I spent the session talking about her daughter, whom I also knew well and who was a brilliant and ambitious student in school. I spoke to her about the values she had instilled in her daughter and how she was respectful to her mother, but I also asked her about her own adolescence and whether she had ever had a crush on a boy. After much hesitation she told me that she had had a crush on a neighbour for years and would make sure she went out into the street to take out the garbage when she knew he would be able to see her. We started to talk about the difficulty of having so many restraints in Afghanistan and having to live in fear, and then I slowly brought the conversation back to her daughter and whether she felt it was good to make her have to live in fear or whether it would be best to encourage her daughter to talk to her and be open with her so that she could guide her young daughter to make the right choices as she grew into a woman. I therefore challenged the woman's belief and did not align with her position against the daughter. After this session we had a few sessions with the mother and daughter together where they were able to talk openly about growing up in the Afghani community in London and the dos and don'ts, and the mother was extremely supportive of her daughter, who opened up more and more to her mother.

If I had not had the confidence to challenge this mother's belief system, I would not have been able to help her and her daughter. I believe being confident about your own culture and beliefs and being able to be self-reflexive is essential in having the skill to engage with families from other cultures, and not accepting everything they bring as the truth.

According to Owusu-Bempah (2002), psychotherapy, which often aims to increase self-awareness and self-efficacy, necessitates an understanding of the self; this can be enriched by learning how other cultures perceive the self. The Western notion of a differentiated autonomous self is alien to most cultures. Moghaddam (1993) goes so far as to question whether it is useful to export Western clinical services to traditional collectivist societies where there already exist traditional supportive psychologies. In other words, psychotherapy as practised in the West is virtually unknown and perhaps unnecessary in the majority of world cultures. In Middle Eastern countries, for example, people are in general very involved with each other's lives, and the elders often offer guidance and advice to family members and friends. There is therefore a great deal of community support, and one does not usually feel isolated or have the need to seek outsider help in the way Westerners seek expert help and support. There is no such thing as personal space, and people in general get involved in your life on a daily basis. One time I was in Iran with my daughter, then aged four. She was hot and asked to take her jacket off; however, within minutes I had to put her jacket back on again as every passer-by commented on it being cold and 'why is this child without a jacket?!'

Maitra (1996) warns that 'practice, if based on Western (professional) views of "normal" family function or child-rearing, can and does result in serious errors in assessment and makes therapeutic interventions useless if not abusive in themselves' (p. 288). In her interview, Sophie said that she could never get refugee parents to agree to bring their children, whereas I have always been able to do family work after a trustful relationship has been built. This makes me think of a couple of Farsi-speaking families I have seen with non-Farsi-speaking professionals who have not wanted to bring their children to the sessions and who later told me they were afraid my colleague would encourage the children to be more 'Western' and support them in their demands and requests which went against our culture. Many times, I have seen colleagues of mine, who have had training in cultural sensitivity, make assessments of situations based on their own values; one example is saying that an Arab father was a bad father because he did not engage with his child through playing with him on the floor. The father in question was a very caring father and did other things for his child, and I had to challenge my colleague's assessment of him and explain that not all fathers, especially in the Middle Eastern cultures, play with their children on the floor. These situations occur often, and in my view, they occur because we do not want to be aware of our own, perhaps, unconscious biases and to see how we judge difference rather than be curious about it.

My interviews show that a competent cross-cultural ethnic practitioner should have the cultural knowledge and linguistic skills to deliver effective interventions to members of that culture. Owusu-Bempah (2002) argues, however, that this is not an absolute requirement for an effective therapeutic outcome. According to him, although the therapist may be knowledgeable about a particular culture or language, other factors, such as social class, may also militate against therapeutic effectiveness; I agree with this viewpoint, especially in the Iranian society, which is very class based and people from different classes do not often mix. Furthermore, the sharing of ethnicity by professionals and their clients does not always exclude the intrusion of stereotypes and assuming you know the culture. I was working with an Iranian man a couple of years ago who was from Ahvaz, which is on the border of Iraq. Being Iranian like him, I mistakenly assumed that I knew his culture and I was soon corrected by him as he explained to me that in that area of Iran, they are mostly Arabic speaking and that their culture is more Arabic than Persian. Furthermore, they have a tribal culture which is very different to a big city such as Tehran; I therefore learned that even though we were both from the same country, it did not necessarily mean we shared the same culture.

This leads me to think about what Krause (2002) suggests in working cross-culturally; she says the clinician needs to take two steps in order to work with uncertainty of other cultures and risk in as safe and ethical a way as possible. The first step is to assume coherence, to join with our clients and attune to their meanings. The second step is to examine our own assumptions in relation to the material with which we are presented, and it is in acting on this self-reflection that we need to take risks to find out more. I believe we need to genuinely want to understand our clients and what they mean from their own perspective; and because we are different from them, we can only do so by being aware of our own views; this is why the notion of self-reflexivity in systemic theory is so essential in engaging in cross-cultural therapeutic work. Furthermore, a big part of our cultural inheritance and what influences our beliefs and values is implicit and so, as therapists, we have to be ready to deal with a constant tension of sameness and difference between our own cultural influences and those of our clients. I agree with Bertrando (2012) when he suggests that the aim of the therapist is not to reach a sense of sameness with the client through relativising one's own culture but to be present and curious as 'the other' to family members and trying to find a mutual process with the family of a sense of shared humanity.

I especially like the way in which Avigad and Pooley (2002: 83) speak about working with refugees:

> When working with refugee families, we—both therapists and clients alike— are strangers in foreign lands. We need to find a world where we can stand together as we try to create a shared language and understanding, where we can work together on a shared belief system about the possibilities of relationship and find a way of communicating that makes sense to us both.

Khan (2002) sees therapy as an exchange of interpretation rather than knowledge between therapist and client. She therefore says that the very self and identity of the therapist, both personal and professional, become tools for engaging in the therapeutic relationship. This means the therapist having constant conversations with themselves as to how he/she/they are participating in the relationship with the client, as well as conversations with the client to get feedback about the process of therapy and the therapeutic relationship. Although in principle I agree with Khan, my concern would be that knowing the Iranian culture, as well as the Kurdish and Afghani cultures, I doubt that anyone would give anything but good feedback to their therapist.

Secrecy of Families and Presumptions of Professionals

One aspect which complicates engaging in a therapeutic relationship with refugees is that refugees and asylum seekers often present stories to the outside world that are highly selective; they consciously construct a shielding narrative to survive. This means that entering the lives of refugees, there is a type of functional distrust that maintains a level of integrity but allows the refugee the best chance of survival in a potentially hostile encounter, very similar to the functional aspects of silence which I have discovered.

Another important aspect of working with families from other cultures is the danger of the professional assuming he/she knows and therefore not being curious enough or judging a complaint as psychosomatic when it is not. Ahlberg (2007) gives a very touching example of this when she writes about a Kurdish woman who sought medical help, in Norway, for consistent vaginal discharge and abdominal pain from having been 'burnt inside', as she put it. She was rejected as a mentally unstable person by an unsuspecting Norwegian medical practitioner who could not imagine torture of the genitals being probed with electrical rods.

Cultural Curiosity and Self-Reflexivity

It is clear that being culturally sensitive is extremely important and valued in the field of family therapy; however, being culturally sensitive is not enough, and we need a better understanding of the challenges the multi-cultural context poses for practising therapists. Rober (2012) says that one challenge could, for example, be the tension a family therapist may feel between his/her/their cultural sensitivity and his/her/their resistance to patriarchal gender practices when working with families for which traditional patriarchal gender roles are the cultural norm. I agree with Rober when he says that we need deeper reflection about the complexity of such issues and that if the therapist only has the idea of being culturally sensitive to hold on to, the risk is that, in his/her/their resolution to respect others, they would be so careful not to offend that this may result in a kind of passivity in which the therapist disappears and is absent rather than respectful. It is therefore essential to reflect deeper on culture in family therapy practice, and especially on ways to deal through reflexivity with difference and sameness in the construction of intercultural therapeutic relationships (Malik and Krause, 2005).

Campbell (2012) says that we need to explore important aspects of the dialogue process in order to create dialogue between people who have different experiences based on race and culture. He explains that each participant feels safe in a dialogue, and that this feeling of safeness is when they believe their conversational partner acknowledges and respects the reasons they are living their lives as they are. According to Campbell, we do not need to fully understand the other's experience; the dialogues being dynamic, we become more or less respectful during conversation. Across the years there have been many discussions about the need to hold expertise alongside practices of not-knowing. Mason (1993) has spoken about the position of 'authoritative doubt', while Larner (2000) has explored the paradox of 'knowing not to know'. In my opinion more thought needs to be given to the significance of therapists' failure to know. This makes me think of Akbar, who said that when he went to see a therapist, he would have had to spend so long educating her about Afghanistan, our history, our society, our culture and so forth that he decided not to go back.

According to Bertrando (2012), therapists' and patients' emotions are a part of any therapeutic interaction and are moulded during the course of it; this is similar to what Daniel (2012) calls 'a meeting place' where, as therapists, we reflect on the feedback we receive about ourselves as cultural/gendered beings, whereby we develop. I suppose the only reservation I have about this is that often Middle Eastern clients do not give feedback to their therapist for cultural reasons. One of the reasons is that they have a lot of respect for the professional 'expert' and would not allow themselves to challenge or question anything they said openly and also because they would not want to lose face and make it look like the therapist was unable to be helpful to them. I have known Middle Eastern families who kept on seeing the same therapist for months without really connecting or feeling they were being helped. When I asked why they did not stop the therapy they said they did not want to question the GP's choice to send them to that therapist and they also did not want to disrespect the therapist by not going. In the end, they were referred to me by their therapists, who decided they may be better helped by someone from their own culture, or familiar with their culture.

Afuape (2011) asserts that an important part of joint action and becoming an 'us' is relational reflexivity defined by Burnham (2005) as the mutual to-ing and fro-ing between the therapist and client in their attempt to make the relationship helpful to the client. She goes on to say that it is important that clients have the power to initiate change in the therapeutic relationship. Afuape proceeds to talk about the importance of relational responsivity in the therapeutic relationship. Resonances and responsivity refer to ways in which we are changed by what we hear in therapy. According to Afuape, the consequences and responsibilities for the therapist who respects and connects to the client's reality are enormous. She writes that when we are relationally responsive to others, we allow ourselves to be ethically answerable to them. 'Therapy in this way', Afuape says, 'Involves an opening of hearts with a willingness on the part of the therapist to have their hearts broken' (p. 120). Indeed, I have had my heart broken many times in working with refugees as I have lived through their suffering with them and helped them to see the light at the end of the tunnel, almost holding their hand as we walked in the darkness towards the light.

I like Turner's (2007) model of intervention with refugees, which is in three phases. In the first phase, Turner emphasises his work with the refugee client on achieving safety (legal status, etc.). I agree with him when he says that this is essential because it is hard to undertake more in-depth therapy until these basic aspects have been achieved; indeed, unless the refugee feels safe he/she/they cannot begin to engage in a therapeutic relationship. Phase two is moving on to therapy, although it is always probable that one may have to go back to phase one every now and again when problems emerge. To me, this is a very difficult reality whereby it is crucial that the therapist is there for the patient not only in the therapeutic setting but is alongside them in helping them with their problems with housing, benefits, schools and so forth. In phase three, the emphasis is on integration and adaptation. Throughout this process, creating a safe and trustful relationship with the refugee is a key factor.

Sometimes important information will be missed or underestimated because of the differences between patient and therapist, but also, as I have said before, I believe because the patients will not trust the therapist enough to tell them every-thing. This may result in the patient assuming that the therapist is unable to listen to their real problems or is not interested or, worse still, does not believe the patient's story. I agree with Alayarian (2007) when she says that the development of the capacity to think without fear again, to be curious and to get involved in therapy, depends on the refugee's experience of being listened to and held in mind and knowing that the therapist is attentive and interested in what they present. In thinking about Sophie's interview when she talks about her colleagues' attitudes towards refugee families ('they should be grateful'), I can only imagine how dif-ficult it must be for the refugee clients to feel heard and understood by them. To this I would like to add the importance of the therapist being empathetic and not hesitating to show the empathy to the refugee. I do not believe that having a neu-tral stance is helpful when working with refugees; they need to see and feel the connectedness and empathy of the therapist.

In writing the previous paragraph, I am reminded of a powerful experience I had recently. My English-speaking colleague and I were seeing an Afghani refu-gee together, and we had been working together for a year. In the sessions, I would act as both co-therapist and interpreter. In one of the sessions, the Afghani man was showing us horrific pictures of people being hung by the Taliban in Afghanistan; picture after picture I passed on to my colleague and explained the reasons given for each execution (feeling the distress rise in me). At one point, he gave me a picture of a pregnant woman who had been hung for infidelity, and as I showed my colleague I broke down in tears and cried with pain at the sight of my fellow men and women being killed on a daily basis (I am also of Afghani descent). The client sat in silence and cried with me and just looked at me with a warm smile through his tears. I apologised, and he held up his hand to stop me and thanked me and said he now knew that I truly was one with him, that I too am an Afghani (if only in part) who loves my country. He said he had believed up until then that because I had lived in Europe for so many years, I was no longer really able to understand where he was coming from and how he longed for his country and the pain he feels at the injustice happening back home. After this session, my colleague and I both noticed how our sessions changed and how much more he shared with us from his traumatic past experiences, which helped our work together move forward faster and better, with no unsaid stories, secrecy or mistrust. I think a therapist from a different cultural context can show compassionate emotions so that an understanding of anguish can be conveyed as a way of starting to build some trust.

Consistency of Care

Like the refugees I interviewed, many of my patients have complained about having to change therapists without warning and without any explanation. Furthermore, the care given seems to often be sporadic when these patients need consistency and containment; in the context of such difficulties, seeing a therapist once a month is not enough and often leaves the patient feeling even more vulnerable.

To me, Pocock (2012) says something essential when working with any client, but I believe especially when working with refugees, which is that the therapeutic encounter depends on whether a new attachment can be made between family members and therapist. To my mind, creating this attachment can help to restore the inner strength of the person and to find their somewhat lost identity. One cannot create this attachment if one sees the therapist with long intervals and the damage is great when the therapist disappears and a new therapist comes along. Refugees take so long to build a trusting relationship and they have already experienced so much loss that when their therapist suddenly changes, they often feel rejected and deeply hurt. Varvin (1998) claims that trauma puts the subject in a position in which he will re-experience not only the helplessness he felt as a child but also the strength and caring received. Hence, recovery from the traumatic experience is dependent on gaining access to the same level of internalised object relationship at which the damage revealed itself, to provide victims with a new beginning. According to Varvin and Hauff (1998), the main purpose of therapy for severely traumatised patients who tend to be incapable of accepting the possibility of a future for themselves is to get their internal clock started again so that the trauma can be integrated as part of the past. I believe this is why it is so crucial to talk about the past and acknowledge refugees' past lives, both positive and negative; unless we take time to do this, we cannot help the patient to see the trauma as part of the past as it has not been worked through. In doing this work with the traumatised patient we need to make them feel safe and contained so they feel less helpless.

References

Afuape, T. (2011), *Power, Resistance and Liberations in Therapy with Survivors of Trauma, to Have Our Hearts Broken*. London: Routledge Publications.

Ahlberg, N. (2007), *'No Five Fingers Are Alike' What Exiled Kurdish Women in Therapy Told Me*. London: Karnac Books Ltd.

Alayarian, Aida. (2007), Trauma, Resilience and Creativity. In *Resilience, Suffering and Creativity*. London: KarnacBooks Ltd.

Avigad, J. & Pooley, J. (2002), Strangers in Foreign Lands. In B. Mason and A. Sawyerr (eds.), *Exploring the Unsaid, Creativity, Risks and Dilemmas in Working Cross-Culturally*. London: Karnac.

Beeman, W.O. (1976), Status, Style and Strategy in Iranian Interaction. *Anthropological Linguistics*, 18: 305–322.

Beeman, W.O. (1986), *Language, Status and Power in Iran*. Bloomington: Indiana University Press.

Bertrando, P. (2012), Cultural and Family Ethos in Systemic Therapy. In B. Krause (ed.), *Culture and Reflexivity in Systemic Psychotherapy, Mutual Perspective*. London: Karnac.

Bowen, M. (1978), *Family Therapy in Clinical Practice*. New York: Jason Aronson.

Burnham, J. (2005), Relational Reflexivity: A Tool for Socially Constructing Therapeutic Relationships. In C. Flaskas, B. Maon and A. Perlesz (eds.), *The Space Between: Experience, Context and Process in the Therapeutic Relationship*. London: Karnac Books.

Campbell, D. (2012), Can We Tolerate the Relationships That Race Compels? In B. Krause (ed.), *Culture and Reflexivity in Systemic Psychotherapy, Mutual Perspectives*. London: Karnac (Placeholder1).

Daniel, G. (2012), With an Exile's Eye: Developing Positions of Cultural Reflexivity (with a Bit of Help from Feminism). In B. Krause (ed.), *Culture and Reflexivity in Systemic Psychotherapy, Mutual Perspectives*. London: Karnac.

Khan, S. (2002), Visible Differences: Individual and Collective Risk-Taking in Working Cross-Culturally. In B. Mason and A. Sawyerr (eds.), *Exploring the Unsaid; Creativity, Risks and Dilemmas in Working Cross-Culturally*. London: Karnac.

Krause, B. (2002), Uncertainty, Risk-Taking and Ethics in Therapy. In B. Mason and A. Sawyer (eds.), *Exploring the Unsaid*. London: Karnac.

Larner, G. (2000), Towards a Common Ground in Psychoanalysis and Family Therapy: On Knowing Not to Know. *Journal of Family Therapy*, 22: 61–82.

Maitra, B. (1996), Child Abuse: A Universal 'Diagnostic' Category? The Implication of Culture in Definition and Assessment. *International Journal of Social Psychiatry*, 42: 287–304.

Malik, R. & Krause, B. (2005), Before and Beyond Words: Embodiment and Intercultural Therapeutic Relationships in Family Therapy. In C. Flaskas, B. Mason and A.P. Perlesz (eds.), *The Space Between: Experience, Context and Process in the Therapeutic Relationship*. London: Karnac, pp. 95–110.

Mason, B. (1993), Towards Positions of safe Uncertainty. *Human Systems*, 4: 189–200.

Moghaddam, F. (1993), Traditional and Modern Psychologies in Competing Cultural Systems: Lessons from Iran 1978–1981. In U. Kim and J.W. Berry (eds.), *Indigenous Psychologies: Research and Experience in Cultural Context*. London: Sage, pp. 104–117.

Owusu-Bempah, K. (2002), Culture, Self, and Cross-Ethnic Therapy. In B. Mason and A. Sawyerr (eds.), *Exploring the Unsaid, Creativity, Risks and Dilemmas in Working Cross-Culturally*. London: Karnac.

Papadopoulos, R.K. (1999), Storied Community as Secure Base. *The British Journal of Psychotherapy*, 15: 322–332.

Papadopoulos, R.K. (April 2001), Refugees, Therapists and Trauma: Systemic Reflections. *Context*, 54.

Papadopoulos, R.K. & Hulme, V. (2002), Transient Familiar Others. Uninvited Persons in Psychotherapy with Refugees. In R.K. Papadopoulos (ed.), *Therapeutic Care for Refugees. No Place Like Home*. London: Karnac, Tavistock Clinic Series.

Pocock, D. (2012), Objectification, Recognition and the Intersubjective Continuum. In K. Flaskas (ed.), *Culture and Reflexivity in Systemic Psychotherapy, Mutual Perspectives.* London: Karnac.

Rober, P. (2012), The Challenge of Writing about Culture and Family Therapy Practice. In I.B. Krause (ed.), *Culture and Reflexivity in Systemic Therapy, Mutual Perspectives.* London: Karnac.

Turner, S. (2007), Memory for Trauma. In A. Alayarian (ed.), *Resilience, Suffering and Creativity: The Work of the Refugee Therapy Centre.* London: Karnac.

Varvin, S. (April 1998), Psychoanalytic Psychotherapy with Traumatised Refugees. Integration, Symbolisation and Mourning. *American Journal of Psychotherapy*, 52(1).

Varvin, S. & Hauff, E. (1998), Psychoanalytically Oriented Psychotherapy with Torture Victims. In I. Jaranson and J.M. Popkin (eds.), *Caring for Victims of Torture.* Washington, DC: American Psychiatric Press, pp. 117–130.

Voulgaridou, M.G., Papadopoulos, R.K. & Tomaras, V. (2006), Working with Refugee Families in Greece: Systemic Considerations. *Journal of Family Therapy*, 28: 200–220.

Woodcock, J. (1995), Healing Rituals with Families in Exile. *Journal of Family Therapy*, 17: 397–409.

Chapter 7

Working with Refugees and Refugee Families

Being given the opportunity to build a trusting and stable therapeutic relationship is the first step in building the refugee's sense of self again and, with the new short-term therapies put in place by Mental Health Services, when the refugee is being forced to 'give up' such an important therapeutic relationship after 6–12 sessions, it can feel almost like a re-traumatisation which hinders them from moving on. This is especially the case when refugees have not been forewarned or consulted before the rupture of the therapeutic relationship; the refugee is left feeling helpless, unheard and abandoned. I have even heard some refugee clients blame themselves for perhaps having been too needy and therefore overwhelming the therapist. It is therefore important for the therapist to be very clear about the number of sessions their service allows them to offer the refugee/asylum seeker and to also take time to explore what the separation from the therapist may mean to them and to begin to have these conversations from the beginning so that the patient does not feel that the therapy has come to an end abruptly. Making sure that the therapy comes to an end in a gentle and collaborative way and enabling the client to have some sense of control and agency can thus be healing instead of re-traumatising.

Through my interviews and my work as a family therapist, I have come to understand that in order to help refugees see their traumatic experiences as part of the past, we, as therapists, should not be overly keen to move too quickly towards the future. We must allow the refugee time to mourn the past and to remember over and over again. We must take the position of a non-judgemental witness to their story, their pain, their hopes, and bear witness to the great losses they have suffered. This, I believe, is an important part of the healing process, and unless we take time to do this, we are moving too fast, which can itself be experienced as abusive.

When I work with refugee families who have suffered trauma, I begin by working in parallel, but separately, with each parent. I let them know that what they say to me in their one-on-one session is confidential (unless they are putting themselves or others at risk), and I say that if there are things which come up which I feel it would be helpful to discuss with their spouse and/or the children, we will speak about this and negotiate what to bring up and how. I give them the time

DOI: 10.4324/9781003310716-8

and space to build a trusting relationship where they can begin to open up at their own pace. I take time to listen to their stories, even if they are repeated in each session, and show respect, acceptance and empathy through body language and words. If they only speak about their physical aches and pains, I take time to acknowledge these. Once trust has been established (which can take several months) I begin to introduce psycho-education about trauma and post-traumatic stress disorder (PTSD) and then eye movement desensitisation and reprocessing (EMDR) treatment. This is an important part of the process of building a trustful therapeutic relationship because once I explain trauma and the effects of it on the person, the clients can begin to let go of the shame they feel and the self-blame for the changes they see in themselves. They can begin to feel hope that they will get better and will be able to re-connect to who they really are underneath the trauma. They can finally feel understood in their pain.

Parallel to the work with each parent, I have couple sessions where I help them to remember their past and what they were like before the trauma, back home when they were in charge of their lives. However, I only see the couple together once the couple begins to trust me and know that I can contain the session and make sure it is a safe place for both of them together. The couple sessions are an important part of the work. I try to help the couple to remember why they chose each other, and every time there is a warm look from one to the other or if they use the same word, I emphasise these moments; many times couples have told me that it is often only in their sessions with me that they feel really married again. After a while, this feeling of being married and sharing a story together becomes part of their life again. There are, of course, cases where the couple decide to separate, and in that case I help them to put together an age-appropriate script about the family journey and how they came to the decision to live separately for the children.

I also have family sessions together with the children to begin to talk about the present and past issues they each want to talk about; usually we begin with school problems and subjects which feel safe, and I slowly guide them towards talking about the past and the effect of their adverse experiences on the family dynamics. In the family sessions I must be very careful to respect the hierarchy of the family to demonstrate respect to the father and not challenge him directly in front of the children. I also need to be a bridge between the children and their parents and almost help them re-negotiate boundaries and develop new rules. I try to create a space where each member of the family feels heard and supported and can therefore feel free to express themselves. I often find myself re-framing what the children are saying so that the parents can hear them without getting offended. Likewise, I almost translate what the parents demand from their children in a way which can be listened to and respected by the children and where the parents feel in control. Over time, my role as the bridge between the family members and the different cultures becomes less significant as the family members learn to talk to each other more openly and have less and less need for me to intervene. Sometimes if I feel the parents are too stuck in the past and therefore hinder the children from adapting to their new lives here. I see the parents separately and try to gently challenge some of their beliefs and help them understand that by taking very rigid positions, they often force the child to hide things from them. I help them understand that when in a foreign country with a culture that is so different to theirs, it is better to try to be more curious about their child's lived experiences in school and in the society to be able to guide them rather than to reprimand them. I point out that if you reprimand the child, there is more risk of the child becoming secretive and hiding important things from you. This, in turn, creates a distance between the child and the parents where they each feel they cannot understand or trust each other, thus putting the child at risk. I often use myself in these sessions, as I have brought up my children in a culture that is different to my Persian culture and I was myself brought up in cultures which were different to my parents' culture. In between these sessions I see the children on their own (but only once the parents trust me). It is very important that the parents feel confident in me seeing the children on their own and can therefore encourage their child(ren) to feel comfortable and to use the space to talk about themselves as well as their parents. Sometimes, the rigid position a parent or parents may take with regard to their child's education can go against my own personal beliefs, of course, and that is when I try to become even more curious and attempt to understand where their fear is coming from, because in my experience fear leads to a rigid and inflexible position, and this can escalate if not listened to. I try to dig deep into the origins of a certain belief in their family and culture, and I can then, often, start to gently introduce a slightly more flexible way of thinking and reach a compromise, again by educating the parents about the dangers of being too rigid when one is not living in one's country and is surrounded by other influences.

These various complex levels and contexts of therapeutic work (parents individually, parents together, children separately, and family sessions) need to happen side by side and together so that the family can move out of their trauma and the past and feel more confident and connected in the present. It needs a great deal of patience, as we usually move one step forward and two steps back in the beginning and I have to hold the hope for the family members who are often deflated and depressed. When we have moments of laughter together, I highlight these and celebrate them, marking the moment; when the children are present, these shared moments of laughter are very special because they see their parents interacting in a different and more positive way. I find that the refugee and asylum-seeking families I work with are asking for hope because they often feel so hopeless themselves. I therefore highlight even the slightest positive change in them and let them know that it is these small changes which lead to bigger ones. I comment on their posture and presentation, which I always see change as the therapeutic work progresses, where their growing confidence takes shape in their body. I often notice how some of my female clients begin to wear brighter colours as their mood and mental well-being improve, and I make sure they know I have noticed this. With couples, if I see them sitting closer together and talking (rather than sitting in silence, which they start off doing), I comment on this and they are often surprised as they have not noticed the change themselves because it happens so gradually. After a while, the family members can begin to hold the hope themselves and give each other encouragement and faith in a better future for them as a family.

Creating building blocks in this way requires making sure that the foundations are stable. Without accompanying the refugees in their past, every step of the way, the good and the bad, we cannot start to build anything merely by focusing on their strengths and resilience. My experience tells me that unless each family member's past identity is heard and held in mind, they will find it difficult to be able to work together as a family where they have to show empathy and to compromise. Through the therapist showing empathy and building trust, the family members learn to show their own vulnerabilities in the sessions, as they feel safe enough to do so. Once they feel contained and supported in their vulnerabilities, they begin to feel more confident and can be more thoughtful about their children's needs and able to be more present. This process can take several months, and it is an important journey to make together with the refugee and their family. By listening to their past identities and lives, the therapist can implicitly highlight the person's strengths and gently remind them of who they can be; this is the first step in emphasising the person's strength and resilience without silencing them from showing weakness and suffering.

Many years ago, I was working with an Afghani couple, and I found it heartbreaking to see their and their children's suffering. I was therefore doing everything in my power to help them move on and be positive, emphasising their strengths. However, after a while I realised I was not getting very far and, after receiving advice from a very experienced and dear colleague of mine, Dr Arturo Varchevker, I let go of the present (and future) and travelled back in time with the couple and asked them to tell me what they had not been able to bring with them in their suitcases when they left their home, what they would have wanted to bring along. This seemed to bring about a very positive change in the therapeutic process whereby the couple was able to re-connect with each other as they spoke about their past and shared dreams. We spent many sessions remembering, and I helped them to mourn the past, a process which was essential. It helped them to heal individually and as a couple; it helped them become more confident as parents and to remember how to hold their children in mind again and it helped them to believe in themselves and their future once more.

The effects of trauma on refugee and asylum-seeking families seem to be that they, at times, lack a sense of purpose because of all the losses they have suffered; the literature, as well as my experience from clinical work and from the research interviews point to a loss of one's sense of self. This feeling of loss and despair, alongside other effects of trauma which are the symptoms mentioned in PTSD, often lead to refugees isolating themselves because keeping another person in mind seems too difficult. When considering refugee/asylum-seeking families from Middle Eastern cultures, an important factor which adds to the complexity, is the cultural script of 'not voicing painful things as they just hurt more'.

The silence thus created and adhered to implicitly further isolates the different members of the family and leads to them living parallel lives under the same roof.

The complexity of changes to the family structure as a result of forced migration is another important aspect which needs to be considered. The father usually loses his status as 'head of the family', and this often causes him to distance himself even more from his family because of a sense of uselessness. Furthermore, it is often difficult for children to adapt to their new status or non-status in society, and as they grow up they may have a deep sense of loss because of having mentally and emotionally absent parents and therefore not be able to find an identity through mirroring that of their parents. A child develops through being held in mind by the caregiver, and although all the refugee parents I have worked with have been extremely caring, they have not had the mental capacity to hold their child in mind when their own suffering was too much to bear. In my experience the parents need to be held in mind themselves by the therapist in order, over time, to be able to heal and find their inner self and identity again. We need, in essence, to become attachment figures to the refugee. In my work with refugee families, I make sure they know that they can count on me to help them individually, as a couple and as a family. I help them in their daily lives as well, contacting housing, the job centre, the children's school and any other authority they may need help with. I am essentially their therapist and also their advocate, and this shows my commitment to helping them feel safe enough to move into the present.

Trauma has the effect of creating mistrust within the couple relationship and a sense of blaming, both of the self and the other. Families seem to get stuck in this state of silence and blame, not trusting the other partner to be able to hear or bear witness to their pain. This is why I always begin to work with each of the partners separately; it is also to understand how much they want to share with their partner. Alongside the intricacies within the family system, there are all the added social and political complexities which effect refugee and asylum-seeking families. Complexities such as not knowing the language and culture of the new host country, racism and feeling undermined and unwelcome. This is why I have found it an important part of the therapeutic relationship to become their advocate as well; I find one cannot talk about therapy and re-building relationships within the family system, when they are at risk of losing their benefits for example. It is important to work with the refugee/asylum-seeking family's reality.

The difficulties of working with these levels of complexities are evident from the analysis of my interviews of professionals and service users. Professionals can often feel overwhelmed and de-skilled, and this can cause the refugee to feel unheard, or worse, disbelieved. This then leads to the refugee mistrusting the professional and adds to a negative and unhelpful cycle. The therapeutic relationship may be hampered by language problems, clients withholding information out of respect, lack of trust, shame, numbing or lack of emotional expression, the stigma of mental illness, difficulties communicating with therapists from a different culture and therapists' bias in accepting or understanding cultural language or suggesting culture-specific treatments. When working with refugees it is important to have regular supervision to be able to voice one's own feelings and also get help and support in thinking about ways to help refugee families. Therapists can, at times, feel hopeless too, and supervision is essential in the therapist's self-care.

Cultural matching and language matching seem to be important to consider when working with refugees because it is significant to know where the other comes from, their culture, the context in which they lived, their values, their everyday lives. Working with refugees means working with someone who has been forced to leave all that is dear to him/her/them because of oppression or persecution on the basis of their political and social convictions and beliefs. Unless the therapist knows where they are coming from politically, socially, historically and culturally, it becomes almost impossible for refugees to engage and feel fully understood. Being from a similar culture also helps the patient believe that they are being less judged, and this assists in building a more trusting relationship faster. Having knowledge about the other's culture and background is not always enough, though, and the therapist needs to be aware of the day-to-day difficulties refugees face, whether these are racial, lack of language, looking different, not knowing the ways of the new society and all the other complexities mentioned in this book.

Bearing in mind what has been said earlier about the Middle Eastern culture of keeping things unsaid, how can one engage a family in therapy without disrespecting their culture and somehow move forward despite the resistance to verbalise painful memories and feelings in front of family members whom they wish to protect? In my experience, as I have already said, it is best to work on an individual level with each member of the couple in order to help them remember the past and gain strength from their positive past identities and assets, as well as take time to mourn trauma and the loss, before working with the couple together in order to help rebuild their relationship. The therapist thus functions as a safe link or bridge between the partners and slowly brings their respective narratives together in a way where each is encouraged to hold in mind the other and feels held in mind by their partner. The therapist must be mindful that each family member may be in a different position on the journey to healing and they may be more or less caught up in their mourning. Once the couple feels more stable, the family as a whole can be worked with because then the parents can be helped to give a coherent narrative about the traumas of the past and the loss to their children; they can be safe parents again where they can be containing to their children. I try to reiterate in every individual and couple session how important it is to speak about the past and that even if they don't name things that happened, their soul and their nervous system remembers and that talking about the past can therefore be healing. Having said this, I help the client choose the memories they are okay to share and others which they do not want to share. Some of the tortures they may have been subjected to in prison, for example, are details that do not need to be shared, unless the refugee wants to. This helps the refugee feel more empowered and therefore less afraid; they begin to open up at their pace.

It would seem that time is essential in helping the refugee to heal and short-term therapies and inconsistencies in care are more damaging than helpful. Even though Mental Health Services are focusing on giving short-term therapies, I am afraid there is no 'quick fix' to the sufferings of this clientele, and by taking the right time and using the right method to make positive changes in these families, we would be saving a lot of valuable time and money in the long run, as the second generation would be helped out of their parents' traumas.

I would like to conclude this book by saying that I am forever grateful to the refugees who agreed to be interviewed and provided me with such valuable insight into the refugees' experiences and trauma. Despite having worked with refugees and asylum seekers for so long, I still did not have as much information and understanding of how much they suffered on their journey here, and even in their home country. The interviews allowed me to thoroughly immerse myself into their experiences and get a more in-depth understanding of the impacts of the adversity they experienced. I have noticed that after these interviews, my work with refugees and asylum seekers improved quite dramatically where I could, with the knowledge I had, ask questions that enabled the client to open up more quickly and trust me because they could sense that I had inner knowledge and understanding. I feel the interviews helped me to really gain insight into what refugees go through and how much they suffer, as individuals and also as a family.

Addendum I

Genogram A

Couple No. I: Fatemeh and Mahdi

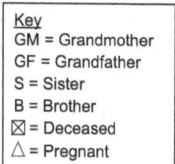

Key
GM = Grandmother
GF = Grandfather
S = Sister
B = Brother
⊠ = Deceased
△ = Pregnant

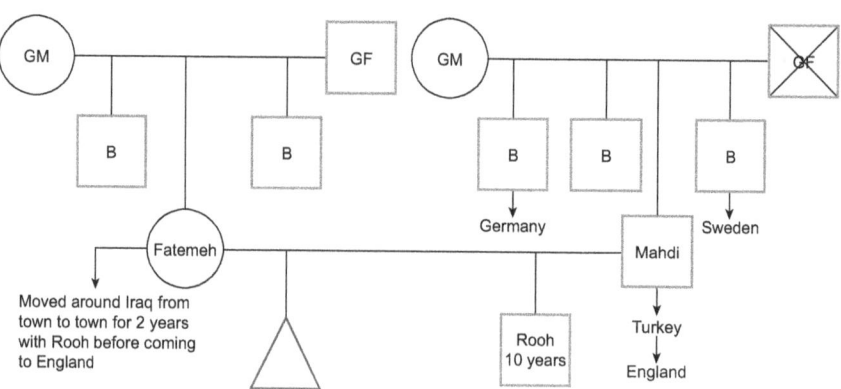

Genogram B

Couple No. 2: Tina and Hamed

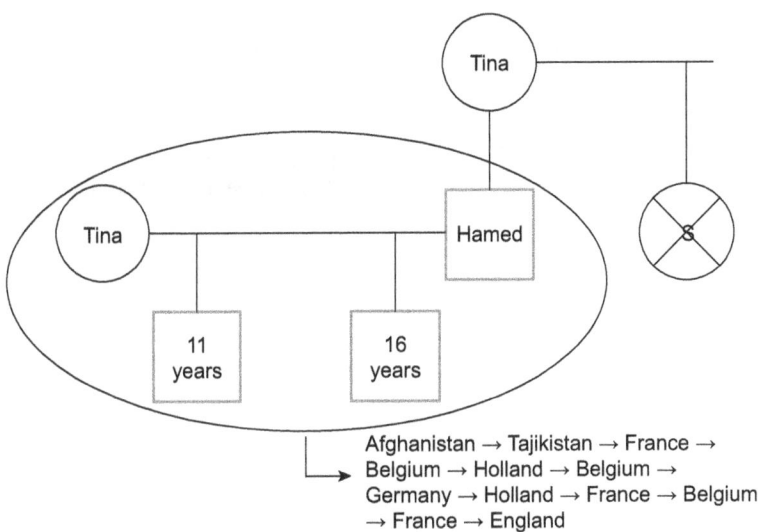

Afghanistan → Tajikistan → France → Belgium → Holland → Belgium → Germany → Holland → France → Belgium → France → England

Genogram C

Couple No. 3: Pooneh and Siavash

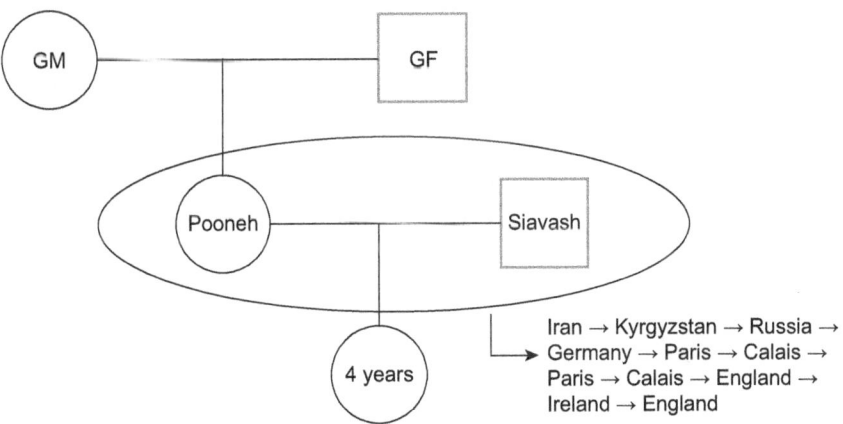

Iran → Kyrgyzstan → Russia → Germany → Paris → Calais → Paris → Calais → England → Ireland → England

Genogram D

Couple No. 4: Nadia and Akbar

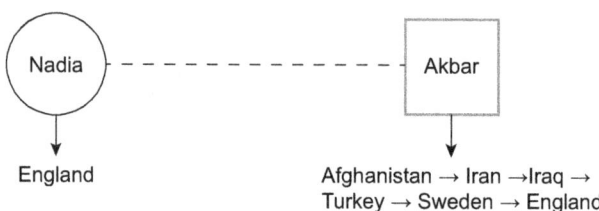

Addendum 2

This is one of my writings which helped me to heal (two years after leaving Iran):

I remember sitting on a stone, looking at the land I belonged to. Every leaf on the trees seemed to be a part of my sad soul and body. The quiet, chilly breeze was like the freezing blood rushing through the worn-out veins inside of me.

The thought of leaving all this beauty brought the sweat to my wrinkled forehead. My eyes were like two big, dark and stormy oceans, refusing the sun. My soul felt like an old tree at Christmas, with all that white, heavy snow burdening upon its back. Oh, I was that tree alright, waiting patiently for someone, some miracle to come and sweep off the snow, far, far away where I would never be able to see it again.

A minute later, the clouds crouched upon the sun, as it immediately surrendered to them, and it rained. It felt so good to know that the skies were sympathising with me. It seemed as if they were trying to make the pool of tears inside of me pour out and wash away the sadness. But even that pool has been covered up with dirt and unmovable soil.

I felt just then the way smokers say they feel about cigarettes. First you enjoy the secrecy of the mysterious smoke, seeking its way through your body, and then, when you're still not ready to give up the pleasure, you find the ashes cooling off in the dirty ash tray.

By now the cool rain had dampened my darkened skin, whilst my inside remained thirsty, and I knew that I would never be able to help it.

As the rain stopped and the birds began to sing once more, memories rushed back and mixed with reality. I wanted to wipe away the present and treasure the past, but that was only wishful thinking. I knew I had to leave my friends, country, my life behind and perhaps never return to it again.

My eyes looked at the calm surrounding me, trying to imprison its beauty. 'This will be my last look', I told myself. I felt so strange just then, so proud of belonging to that peculiar nature.

Yes, I loved my country, and still do, though my conscious tells me that I should put aside its memories and lock them up in the attic of my mind.

I shall never forget it—the past.

Index